Protein engineering of human chorionic antigen

Summary

1- The concentration of intact human chorionic gonadotropin (hCG) and free β subunit (hCGβ) in sera and tissues of patients with gynecologic cancers was determined by radioimmunoassay. Intact hCG and free hCGβ levels were found to be elevated above the reference value (5mIU/ml) in sera of 50% of patients with epithelial ovarian cancer and in sera of 44% of patients with endometrial cancer. The sera intact hCG and free hCGβ levels were significantly higher in malignant then in non-malignant gynecologic tumors ($P<0.05$). Elevation intact hCG and free hCGβ above 5mIU/ml in tissues was found in 100% of patients with epithelial ovarian and endometrial cancers.

2- The characteristics of the binding of ^{125}I-hCG to hCG receptor in ovarian and uterine tumors homogenates were investigated using the radio receptor assay (RRA). Different factors affecting this binding were studied and the result showed that the maximum binding was achieved by using 500 and 700 µg protein of ovarian and uterine homogenate respectively, 17 and 4 Pmol of ^{125}I-hCG concentration for ovarian and uterine tumors respectively, pH(7-7.4) for both tumors. Association kinetic studies of the binding reaction revealed the time and temperature dependency. The ^{125}I-hCG binding to the hCG receptor was specifically displaced by low concentration of unlabeled hCG and LH, where IC_{50} was 2.4ng for hCG and 4ng for LH. The RRA appeared that homogenates of malignant ovarian tumor have a specific hCG-binding activity 2 fold higher than that of homogenates of benign.

Endometrial cancer homogenates have binding activity lower than that in malignant and benign ovarian tumors.

3-Method was developed for the purification of hCG receptor from detergent soluble membranes extracts of epithelial ovarian cancer by gel filtration chromatography using Sepharose CL-6B column (1.5 x 87cm) and affinity chromatography using hCG-Sepharose affinity column (2 x 8cm). The purification fold was 8,538 fold. Physicochemical properties of purified hCG receptor were investigated and the

results showed that the Mw 204 KD and the stock's radius 54^0A under non reducing conditions, while the reducing conditions showed three protein component with Mw 80, 350 D, 53,703D, 42,657D respectively, PI 6.4, carbohydrate content 8%. Binding studies demonstrated that the purified hCG receptor retained all the specific binding characterized expected for the hCG receptor. Association kinetic indicated the pseudo first order kinetic of the binding of ^{125}I-hCG to hCG-R, while the kinetic of dissociation was biphasic and characterized by an initial rapid phase followed by a much slower rate of dissociation. The Hill-plot data (n-1) indicated that there was no cooperation between the hCG –R binding sites.

4-The carcinoembryonic antigen (CEA) was investigated in the sera and tissues of patients with ovarian and uterine tumors. The results revealed a slightly elevation of levels of CEA above the reference value (5ng/ml) in the sear of 33% of patients with endometrial cancer and in 43% of patients with epithelial ovarian cancer. CEA immunoreactivities were significantly higher in malignant ovarian homogenates than in corresponding sera samples while not significantly elevated in malignant uterine tissues.

5-Serum LDH, total ALP, and HSAP activity were measured in ovarian and uterine tumors. The LDH activity was higher in patients with epithelial ovarian and endometrial cancers than those of healthy individuals but not statistical significant. The electrophoresis analysis of LDH isoenzymes showed extra band for serum of epithelial ovarian cancer. Total AIP and HSAP activity in the sera of cancer patients were significantly higher than in normal individuals.

6-The elements (copper, zinc, calcium) concentration were measured in the sera of patients with ovarian and uterine tumors. The results revealed an increment in the concentration of zinc in patients with ovarian and endometrial cancer rather than control group, while copper and calcium concentration did not alter in cancer investigated patients

LIST of ABBREVIATIONS

AFP	Alpha –Fetoprotein
ALP	Alkaline phosphatase
B	Bound
BSA	Bovine serum albumin
CA_{125}	Carbohydrate antigen 125
CA_{15-3}	Carbohydrate antigen 15-3
CA_{19-9}	Carbohydrate antigen 19-9
cAMP	3',5' –cyclic adenosine mono phosphate
CD	Circular dichroism
cDNA	Complementary DNA
CNS	Central nervous system
CPM	Counts per minute
CSF	Cerebrospinal fluid
CT	Computed tomography
CTP	Carboxy terminal polypeptide
DNA	Deoxy ribonucleic acid
D	Dalton
EDTA	Ethylene diamine tetra acetic acid
EGF	Epidermal growth factor
ERT	Estrogen replacement therapy
F	Free
FIGO	International federation of gynecology and oncology
FSH	Follicle –stimulating hormone
GTD	Gestational trophoblastic disease
hCG	Human chorionic gonadotropin
hCGβ	β Subunit of human chorionic gonadotropin
hCGα	α Subunit of human chorionic gonadotropin
hCGβcf	Beta –core fragment of hCG
HCG-R	hCG receptor
HSAP	Heat stable alkaline phosphatase
LDH	Lactate dehydrogenase
LH	Luteinzing hormone
LRR	Leucine rich repeats
LSA	Lipid associated sialic acid

MAB	Mono clonal antibodies
MAD	multi wavelength anamalous diffraction
MCA	Mucin like cancer antigen
M-CSF	Macrophage clonny stimulating factor
mRNA	Massenger ribonucleic acid
NGF	Nerve growth factor
NS	Not significant
NSB	Non specific binding
PDGF-ββ	Platelet –derived growth factor – ββ
PAGE	Poly acrylamide gel electrophoresis
PI	Isoelectric point
P^{53}	Tumor suppressor gene
PLK	Polo –like kinase
PMSF	Phenyl methyl sulfonyl flouride
PTH	Parathyroid hormone
RIA	Radioimmuno assay
RRA	Radio receptor assay
SB	Specific binding
SCC	Squamous cell carcinoma
SDS	Sodium dodecyl sulfate
S-phase	Synthesis phase
TAH –BSO	Total abdominal hysterectomy with bilateral salping – oophorectomy
TEMED	N.N,N,N-tetra methyl ethylene diamine
TGF-β	Tumor growth factor - β
TSH	Thyroid –stimulating hormone
UV	Ultra –violet
WGA	Wheat germ agglutinin

Contents

Subject		Page No.
List of Abbreviation		
Summary		
Contents		
ChapterOne: Introduction		
1.1	Gynecologic cancers	1
1.2	Endometrial cancer	1
1.2.1	Histology	2
1.2.2	Etiology	4
1.2.3	Clinical evaluation and treatment	4
1.3	Epithelial ovarian cancer	6
1.3.1	Histology	7
1.3.2	Etiology	8
1.3.3	Clinical evaluation and treatment	8
1.4	Tumor markers in Gynecologic cancers	10
1.4.1	Antigenic markers	11
	Squamous cell carcinoma (SCC) antigen	11
	Lipid associated sialic acid (LsA)	11
	CA-125	11
	Other antigens defined by monoclonal antibodies	12
	Carcinoembryonic antigen (CEA)	12
1.4.2	Genomic markers	13
1.4.3	Enzymatic markers	13
1.4.4	Hormonal markers	14
1.4.4.1	Human chorionic gonadotropin (hCG)	14
A-	Chemical structure of hCG	15
B-	Molecular forms of hCG	17
	Intact hCG	17
	Free hCGβ	18
	Free hCGα	18
	Beta – Core fragment of hCGβ (hCGβcf)	18
	Nicked hCG (hCGn or hCGβn)	18
C-	Production and metabolism of hCG	19
D-	Clinical use of hCG determinations	19
	Diagnosis of pregnancy and related disorders	19
	Placental and testicular trophoblastic tumors	20
	Nontrophoblastic tumors	20
	a- blood studies	21
	b- urine studies	21
	c- effusion fluids studies	21
	d- tissues studies	22
E-	Determination methods of hCG	23

		Biological methods	23
		a- In vivo methods	23
		b- In vitro methods	23
		Binding methods	23
		a- competitive immuno procedures	23
		b- non- competitive immuno procedures	24
1.5		Human chrionic gonadotropin receptor (hCG-R)	25
1.5.1		Structure of the hCG-R and the nature of hormone – Receptor Introduction	26
1.5.2		The role of hCG-R nongonadal tissue and tumor tissue	30
		The aim of the work	32

Chapter Two: Human Chorionic Gonadotropin in Sera and Tissues of Patients with Gynecologic Cancers

Abstract		33
Introduction		34
Materials and methods		34
2.1	Chemicals	34
2.2	Apparatus	35
2.3	Patients	35
2.4	Collection of specimens and preparation of tissue homogenates	36
2.5	Quantitative measurement of intact hCG and free hCGβ	36
2.6	Estimation of protein contents	38
2.7	Statistical analysis	38
	Results and discussion	38
	Preoperative Data	38
	Postoperative Data	44
	Malignant and non malignant tissues	45

Chapter Three: Development of a Radio Receptor Assay for Detection and Analysis of hCG – Receptor in Benign and Malignant Gynecologic Tumors

Abstract		57
Introduction		58
Materials and methods		59
3.1	Buffer and reagents	59
3.2	Patients and specimens	59
3.3	Binding studies of ^{125}I-hCG with Its receptor in Benign and malignant ovarian and uterine tumors	60
3.3.1	Preliminary test of hCG-R binding	60
3.3.2	The effect of ^{125}I-hCG concentration on the binding	60
3.3.3	The effect of receptor concentration on the binding	61
3.3.4	The effect of pH on the receptor binding	61
3.3.5	Temperature dependency of the binding	61
3.3.6	Time course of receptor binding	62
3.3.7	Stability of receptor homogenate and hormone receptor complex	62
3.3.8	Determination of the equilibrium binding constants of hCG – R	63
3.3.9	Specification of binding and determination of IC_{50} and K_i	63
Results and discussion		64
Membrane preparation		64
Human chorionic gonadotropin receptor in ovarian and uterine tumors		65
Factors effecting the binding of ^{125}I-hCG with Its receptor		67

1-	The effect of ^{125}I-hCG concentration on the binding	67
2-	The effect of receptor concentration on the binding	68
3-	The effect of pH on the receptor binding	69
4-	Temperature dependency of the binding	69
5-	Time course of receptor binding	70
6-	Stability of receptor homogenate and hormone receptor complex	71
7-	Determination of the equilibrium binding constants and maximum binding capacity	72
8-	Specificity of binding	73
Chapter Four: Purification and Characterization of hCG – R from Ovarian Cancer		
Abstract		88
Introduction		89
Materials and methods		90
4.1	Buffers and reagents	90
4.2	Patients and specimens	90
4.3	Protein determination	91
4.4	Binding assay	91
4.5	Purification of hCG-R	91
4.5.1	Gel filtration chromatography on Sepharose CL-6B	91
4.5.2	Affinity chromatography on Sepharose-hCG	92
4.6	Analytical and characterization of purified hCG receptor	93
4.6.1	Determination of the association constant	93
4.6.2	Analysis of purified receptor by conventional PAGE	94
4.6.3	Determination of the molecular weight by SDS-PAGE	95
4.6.4	Determination of the molecular weight and stocks radius by gel filtration chromatography	97
4.6.5	Determination of the isoelectric point (pI) of purified receptor	98
4.6.6	Specificity of binding for purified receptor	99
4.6.7	UV spectrum of hCG, and hCG- receptor complex	99
4.6.8	Stability of crude and purified solubilized receptor	100
4.6.9	Binding kinetics of purified receptor	100
4.6.10	Estimation of hill coefficient (n) of purified receptor	101
Results and discussion		101
Purification of the receptor		101
Analytical and characterization of purified receptor		104
Human chorionic Gonadotropin binding properties of purified receptor		104
Polyacrylamide gel electrophoresis		105
Molecular weight of the purified receptor		106
Isoelectric point (pI) of purified receptor		108
Carbohydrate composition of the purified receptor		108
Human chorionic Gonadotropin binding specificity of purified receptor		109
The UV – spectrum of hCG and of hCG-Receptor complex		110
Stability of purified receptor		111
Kinetic of purified receptor binding and the determination of Hill coefficient		112
Chapter Five: Evaluation of some Biochemical Constituents in Gynecologic Cancers		
Abstract		127
Introduction		128

	Material and methods	130
5.1	CEA, LDH, and ALP kits	130
5.2	Apparatus	131
5.3	Patients and specimens	131
5.4	CEA quantitative measurement	131
5.5	Determination of LDH activity	131
5.6	Analysis of LDH by electrophoresis	133
5.7	Determination of alkaline phosphatase activity (ALP)	134
5.8	Determination of heat stable alkaline phosphatase activity (HSAP)	135
5.9	Determination of the elements (Cu^{++}, Zn^{++}, Ca^{++}) concentrations in the sera of tumor patients	136
Results and discussion		136
Biochemical constituents in ovarian and endometrial cancer patients		136
Copper, zinc, calcium in the sera of ovarian and endometrial cancer patients		139
Conclusions		148
The future work		148
References		150

Chapter One

Introduction

Chapter One

Introduction

1.1 Gynecologic Cancers

The major malignancies of the female reproductive tract are endometrial, cervical, and ovarian cancer (Fig.1). Other gynecologic cancers, such as choriocarcinoma, fallopian tube cancer, vagina cancer, and vulva cancer are rare, but cancers metastasis to these female genitals are more common [1].

Ovarian cancer accounts for 4% of the total cancer in women worldwide. In Iraq, this cancer is the eighth most common malignant neoplasm in women (3.8-4.2% of the total cancer) behind cancer of the breast, non-Hodgkin's lymphoma, brain and other CNS, leukemia, urinary bladder, bronchus and lung, and skin. The number of cases for the period (1992-1997) was 828 [2].

The incidence rates of corpus uteri cancer (95% endometrial) were found to be higher in the richer countries and urban populations; it is the fifth leading cancer in women at these countries [3]. However, there is evidence of some change in the socioeconomic determinants of the disease in developed countries. In Iraq, cancer of corpus uteri accounts for (0.9-2.2%) of the total cancer in women. The number of cases for the period (1992-1997) was 477 [2]. The risk of uterine cancer is low before age 40 years and increases sharply thereafter [4].

Most cancers of the vulva, vagina and cervix are detected relatively early because these organs are easily visualized and assessable for examination by cytology and biopsy [1]. Endometrial cancers are also detected early because they normally heralded by vaginal bleeding. In contrast, cancers of the ovary mostly present at a late stage with widespread intra-abdominal metastases. Ovarian cancer remains the most lethal gynecologic malignancy in women [5].

1.2 Endometrial Cancer

Endometrial cancer is the most common type of the corpus uteri (Fig.1c), constituting about 95% of all malignant lesions of the uterine cavity, while uterine sarcomas accounts for fewer than 5 %[3].

The normal endometrium contains two major components: endometrial stroma and glands. The glandular cell produces cytoplasmic receptors for estradiol and, when stimulated, results in proliferation of glandular epithelium, producing larger and more numerous glands. In the premenopausal cycling endometrium, the maturational effects of progesterone from the corpus leteum counter balance the proliferative influence of estrogen. If conception does not occur, the lining is shed and a new cycle is initiated. When ovulation ceases at menopause, the endometrial becomes quiescent and the glands atrophy. Tumors arising from the glandular epithelium, either de novo or as a result of abnormal estrogenic stimulation; are adenocarinomas[6]. The transition from benign proliferative endometrium to well differentiated adenocarcinoma probably proceeds through several intermediary steps, collectively termed hyperplasia. Hyperplasias are characterized by an overgrowth of the glandular component of the endometrial lining, whereas cancers are defined by the size of the cells, irregular nuclear membranes, coarse chromatin clumping, loss of glandular pattern, increasing nuclear atypia, and mitotic activity[6].

1.2.1 Histology

About 90% of endometrial cancers are endometriosis type (adenocarcinomas), which contain glands similar to those seen in the normal endometrium. These tumors are subclassified by their degree of differentiation into three grades:well (grade I, 50%), moderately (grade II, 35%), and poor differentiated (grade III, 15%). The

International Federation of Gynecology and Oncology (FIGO) grading scheme is based on the growth pattern (relative proportion of glandular and solid areas):less

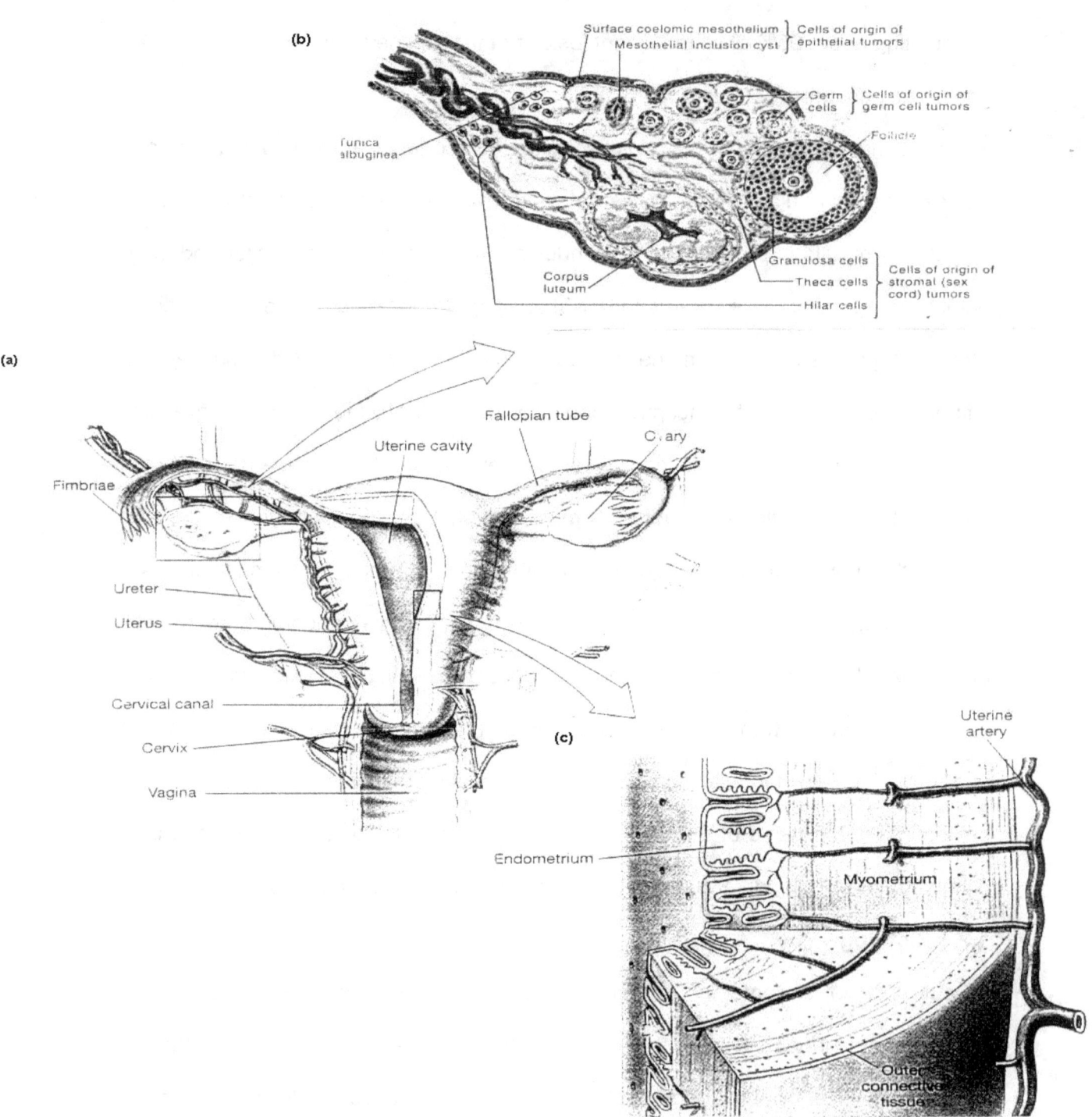

Fig.1 [9] **(a):Female reproduction tract**

(b): Embryologic origins of ovarian cancer.

(c):Tissue layers of uterus

than 5% solid growth is grade I, 6-50% is grade 2, and more than 50% is grade 3[3]. Endometriosis adenocarcinoma accounts for 60-65% of the adenocarcinomas, it is characterized by the disappearance of stroma between abnormal glands, necrosis, and hemorrhage[1].Some typical adenocarcinoma contains areas of squamous metaplasia, which can have a benign or malignant appearance, such tumors are termed adenocarcinoma with squamous differentiation[6].

A variant of endometriosis adenocarcinoma is the villoglandular type, which appears to have more aggressive behavior [7].Uncommon cell types (clear, papillary serous, mucinous, squamous and undifferentiated) account for the remaining 10% of endometrial cancers [6].

1.2.2 Etiology

Endometrial cancer is one of the few malignancies for which the etiology is well understood.Epidemiologic, endocrinologic, and clinical studies have shown that the association between endometrial cancer and most of the identified risk factors can be explained by increased exposure to endogenous or exogenous estrogens.This hypothesis is supported by the increased risk of endometrial cancer (related to obesity, early age at menarche, late age at menopause, low parity or nullparity, certain types of ovarian tumors, history of menstrual disorders, history of infertility, and use of estrogen replacement therapy (ERT) or sequential oral contraceptives).It is also supported by the decreased risk of endometrial cancer (related to the use of combined oral contraceptives, early age at menopause, high parity, and smoking)[4].

Medical conditions such as diabetes, hypertension, and thyroid diseases have been suggested to increase the risk of endometrial cancer, but these finding are not consistent[8].It remains, unclear whether these finding are the result of the association of these medical conditions with obesity or with other biologic mechanisms.

1.2.3 Clinical Evaluation and Treatment

The initial growth phase of most endometrial cancers consists of polyploidy expansion within the endometrial lining. Small areas of necrosis or surface breakdown in the tumor produce abnormal vaginal bleeding. Consequently, the premenopausal women usually present with metrorrhagia, and the older woman has postmenopausal bleeding. Patient with advanced disease may have pelvic pain, bleeding, or bloating[3]. The diagnosis of endometrial can be reliably established by office endometrial biopsy. Dilatation and fractional curettage or hysteroscopy with biopsy may be helpful diagnostic procedures in cases in which out patient biopsy is non diagnostic[1].

The workup on the woman with endometrial cancer should include a physical examination, endometrial biopsy, laboratory studies, and a chest radiograph. Endometrial cancer is typically a disease of women in their sixties and seventies who frequently have coexisting medical problems, so the evaluation should focus on an assessment of operative risk. Additional more sophisticated studies such as proctoscopy, barium enema, ultrasound, computed tomography (CT), or magnetic resonance imaging should be reserved for clinical situations in which advanced disease is suspected[6].

Schematic approach to treatment endometrial cancer is illustrated in (Fig. 2)[6]. Surgical excision of the primary tumor via total abdominal hysterectomy with bilateral salpingo –oophorectomy (TAH-BSO); sometimes accompanied by removal of the pelvic and periaortic lymph nodes; is the mainstay of therapy for endometrial cancer. The selection of additional therapy is based on the result of the staging biopsies of uterine tumors, which was adopted in 1988 (Table 1) by FIGO surgical staging[3].

1.3 Epithelial Ovarian Cancer

The ovary is composed of an outer cortex and an inner medulla. The cortex containing the coelomic surface mesothelium, germ cell (oocytes), specialized hormone producing stroma (granulose and thecal cell), and unspecialized supporting stromal cells. Primary ovarian cancers are classified; according to the structure of the ovary from which the tumor is derived (Fig.1b); into three major categories, epithelial, germ cell, and stromal[9]. The ovary may also be the site of metastasis spread from

Fig.2 Basic treatment strategy for endometrial cancer[6].

Table (1) Surgical staging system for cancer of the uterine body[3].

Stage	Extent
I	**Cancer confined to the corpus**
Ia	Tumor limited to endometrial
Ib	Invasion to less than one half the myometrium
Ic	Invasion to more than one half the myometrium G_1: Well differentiated (≤5% of a nonsquamous or nonmorular solid growth pattern) G_2: Moderately differentiated (6%-50%) G_3: Predominantly solid or undifferentiated
II	**Cancer involves corpus and cervix but does not extend outside the uterus**
IIa	Endocervical glandular involvement only
IIb	Cervical stromal invasion
III	**Cancer extends outside the uterus but not outside the true pelvis**
IIIa	Tumor invades serosa and/or adnexa or positive peritoneal cytology
IIIb	Vaginal metastases
IIIc	Positive pelvic and /or paraaortic nodes

IV	**Cancer extends outside true pelvis or invades bladder or rectal mucosa**
IVa	Tumor invasion of bladder and/or bowel mucosa
IVb	Distant metastases including intra-abdominal and/or inguinal lymph nodes

gynecologic and other tumors. Epithelial ovarian tumors are the most common, accounting for 80-90% of cases[5].

Epithelial ovarian cancers are derived from the coelomic surface mesothelium. During ovulation, the dominant ovarian follicle ruptures, releasing the ovum. To heal the ruptured follicle, surface mesothelial cells proliferate and fill the defect. Inclusion cysts may form and are lined with these mesothelial cells. Over years of repeated ovulation and repeated growth of mesothelia cells, the regulation of this proliferation may become disrupted, allowing the development of tumors (Fig.1b)[9].

Numerous factors can stimulate –or fail to control mesothelial proliferation including growth factors, oncogenes, and tumor suppressor genes[10].

1.3.1 Histology

Epithelial ovarian tumors classified according to cell type, pattern of growth (cystic, solid, and surface), atypia and invasiveness (benign, borderlines, malignant). The ovarian surface epithelium, when involved in neoplastic conditions, often undergoes a mullerian differentiation as a result, it may produce any of the adult epithelia, including tube, endometrial and, endocervical mucosa, singly or in combination. So the histological types of the epithelial tumors are serous, mucinous, endometriosis, clear cell, Brenner, mixed epithelial, undifferentiated, and unclassified[3]. Serous tumors make up about 20% of all benign ovarian tumors and 75% of epithelial ovarian cancers. Malignant serous tumors are usually multicystic, bilateral and resembling fallopian tube epithelium. Serous carcinoma may have a complex mixture of cystic and solid areas with extensive papillations, or they may contain a predominantly solid mass with areas of necrosis and hemorrhage[11]. The second common type of epithelial ovarian cancer is endometriosis tumor (10%) which is histological indistinguishable from endometrial uterine cancer. About 6-10% of epithelial ovarian cancers are mucinous, which characterized by epithelial – mucin producing cell resembling those of the endocervix[9]. Clear cell tumors account for<5% of all primary ovarian cancers. The tumor cell is large and their cytoplasm is clear. These tumors have more aggressive behavior than other epithelial cancers. Brenner tumors, these unusual lesions are though to originate from the ovarian mesothelium despite their urothelial –like transitional cell structure. They are solid and almost benign.

1.3.2 Etiology

Several factors have been associated with an increased risk of epithelial ovarian cancer, while two factors appear to reduce the incidence of this malignancy – pregnancy and use of oral contraceptives – presumably because they suppress ovulation. The risk of epithelial ovarian cancer is high in ovulating nulliparous women, women using of fertility drug, women exposing to hormones (particularly gonadotropins) and carcinogens, such as infectious agents and chemical carcinogens[12].

The large majority of ovarian cancer presumably related to environmental factors, but 5-10% of women with epithelial tumors have a predisposing familial syndrome. Three autosomal dominant syndromes have been identified: site –specific ovarian cancer, hereditary breast –ovarian cancer syndrome, and lynch syndrome II (adenocarcinomas of multiple sites, including breast, ovary, and endometrial, gastrointestinal tract). All three types of familial ovarian cancer develop at a younger age than sporadic ovarian cancer[9].

Other factors, such as obesity, high-fat diet, early menarche, late menopause, single women, may predispose women to develop this malignancy. The hypothesis is that the continual ovulation, uninterrupted by pregnancy may develop the disease[4].

1.3.3 Clinical Evaluation and Treatment

Epithelial ovarian cancer is seldom detected at an early stage; up to 80% of these tumors have metastasized by any of the four routes (peritoneal seeding, lymphatic embolization, direct extension and hematogenous dissemination). The first sign of early ovarian cancer is usually an asymptomatic mass found during a pelvic, rectal, or abdominal examination. A benign tumor or slow- growing cancer may grow quite large and cause abdominal distention and may compress the rectum or bladder, producing constipation, urinary frequency or nocturia. Ovarian tumor occasionally undergoes torsion, resulting in localized pain, nausea, and possibly low fever, and may also cause symptoms of inappropriate estrogen or androgen synthesis[9].

The diagnosis of epithelial ovarian cancer is surgical, usually by a laparotomy, but occasionally at laparoscopy. Ultrasound of adnexal pelvic mass is useful prior to the surgical diagnosis. Most patients with a pelvic mass require ultrasonography, chest radiography, CT, and aspiration of pleural effusion to check for metastases. Mammography should be performed to exclude primary breast cancer[3].

The management of primary epithelial ovarian cancer may be divided into three phases: primary definitive surgery, postoperative adjuvant therapy usually chemotherapy[13], and systematic follow up and reevaluation. The initial surgical procedure (usually TAH-BSO) is used to determine the extent of the disease (staging) and to remove as much gross disease as possible (cytoreduction). In ovarian cancer, metastases adhere superficially to peritoneal surfaces without deep invasion. Therefore, surgical resection of metastasis ovarian cancer is standard care[9]. The tumor must be staged to facilitate planning of adjuvant therapy, the FIGO staging system of 1987 (Table 2)[3] is based on the finding at surgical exploration. Following the cytoreductive surgery or debulking, patients should be treated, generally with chemotherapy and some time with radiation or endocrine therapy[14][15]. The majority of women with advanced epithelial ovarian cancer will ultimately relapse and develop drug-resistant disease.Thus,there is a common need for second-line treatment including cytotoxic drugs,or secondary cytoreductive surgery or palliative surgery[16].

Table (2) Surgical staging system for epithelial ovarian cancers[3].

Stage	Extent (proportion of cases)
I	**Cancer limited to ovaries (15%)**
Ia	Limited to one ovary, no ascites
Ib	Both ovaries involved, no ascites
Ic	Ia or Ib with ascites or positive peritoneal washings
II	**Cancer of one or both ovaries with extension limited to pelvic tissue(15%)**
IIa	Extension to uterus or tubes
IIb	Extension to other pelvic tissues
IIc	IIa or IIb with ascites pr positive peritoneal washings
III	**Cancer involving one or both ovaries with peritoneal implants outside the pelvis and/or positive retroperitoneal or inguinal nodes.Tumor is limited to the true pelvis but with histological proved extension to small bowel or omentum (65%)**
IIIa	Tumor grossly limited to the true pelvis with negative nodes but with histological confirmed microscope seeding of abdominal peritoneal surface
IIIb	Same as IIIa, but abdominal peritoneal implants do not exceed 2 cm in diameter
IIIc	Abdominal implants greater than 2cm in diameter and/or positive retroperitoneal or inguinal lymph nodes
IV	**Distant metastases present (including cytology-positive pleural effusion metastasis liver parenchyma or peripheral superficial lymph nodes(5%).**

1.4 Tumor Markers in Gynecologic Cancers

Tumor markers; which may be considered as any biological aberration that indicates the presence of a tumor; are required for primary diagnosis, histological identification, assessment of the extent of the disease pre- and post operatively, therapy guidance, and early detection of recurrence. Ideally, the tumor marker assessed in serum, or in another body compartment, should accurately reflect the presence and the amount of residual tumor, and should also distinguish benign from malignant disease[17]. In gynecological practice, it is well documented that human chorionic gonadotropin(hCG), alpha-feto protein(AFP), estrogens, and androgens have been contributed greatly to the diagnosis and management of gestational trophoblastic disease, gram cell tumor, and granulose cell tumor, respectively[17][18].

By the introduction of polyclonal and monoclonal antibody technology, variety of tumor carbohydrate associated antigens have been identified as a result of glycosylation changes in the carbohydrate moieties of glycoproteins and glycolipids by tumor cells, some of tumor associated antigens also represent differentiation antigens and receptors that may reexpressed or over expressed[18][19].

1.4.1 Antigenic Markers

1- Squamous Cell Carcinoma (SCC) Antigen: The SCC antigen was described in 1977 as one of 14 subfractions of tumor associated antigen found in human cervical cancer tissue [20]. SCC antigen have been reported to be elevated (>2 ng/ml) in 35% of stage I patients, and increasing to 91% in stage IV for cervical cancer [21][22]. While serum SCC antigen level were increased in 8-29% of endometrial cancer. In vulvar and vaginal squamous cell cancers, the reported frequencies of SCC antigen elevation are lower (42% and 17%, respectively) than in cervical cancer[17].

2- Lipid-Associated Sialic Acid (LSA): Elevated levels of LSA are found in a variety of malignancies, including cancers of the vulva, vaginga, uterus and ovary[18]. Due to its lack of specification, LSA used alone had not been useful in gynecologic cancers.

3- CA-125: Since its first report in 1983[23], CA-125 has been used widely for monitoring epithelial ovarian cancer. Among healthy individuals, 99% will have been serum level <35U/ml[24]. Approximately 85% of ovarian cancer patients have elevated CA-125 level (> 35 U/ml) for all histological types of epithelial ovarian cancers but more frequently for nonmucinous tumors than for mucinous types[25][26]. It is also expressed in cancer of epithelium female reproductive tract[27] and can be detected in 22% of patients with nongynecological cancers (Breast, lung, Colon, Pancreas), also detected in benign gynecological tumors (endometriosis, adenomyosis, ovarian cystadenomas)[28][29].

The low specificity hampers the use of CA-125 as a screening test for ovarian cancer. Combined with pelvic examination and/or ultra sound, the specificity can be increased[30]. The sensitivity of the marker might be also increased by examining peritoneal fluid, where the CA-125 levels are higher than in serum (Cutoff at 200u/ml)[31]. CA-125 is very rarely elevated in endometrial cancer confined to the uterus, whereas elevation is found in 78-100% of cases with extra uterine spread[27].

4- Other Antigens Defined by Monoclonal Antibodies: Following the report of CA-125, a number of monoclonal antibodies such as CA 19-9 and CA 15-3 were developed in colorectal cancer[32], breast cancer[33], ovarian cancer and endometrial cancer[34] as immunnogens, and this explain their lack of specificity.

Various monoclonal antibodies have been raised against epithelial mucin like caner antigen MCA, CA M26, and CA M29. These cancer antigens have been reported in cancers of breast, colon, ovary, endometrial and cervix [35][36], but non of them, either alone or in combination, has been shown to be as useful as CA-125.

Another marker for ovarian cancer is NB/70K which seen to be a marker for all histological types of epithelial ovarian cancer[17]. Serum NB/70K is elevated in all stages of ovarian malignancies, including more than 50% of early stage cases[37][38].

5- Carcinoembryonic Antigen (CEA): This oncofetal protein can be demonstrated in most gynecological cancers immunohistologically, while plasma levels are often too modestly elevated to be useful for diagnosis or for disease monitoring[17]. Slightly elevated plasma CEA levels are seen in approximately 50% of ovarian cancer patients[39][26], and mucinous tumors tend to have highest levels. Measuring CEA with CA-125 and CA19-9 can be useful to differentiate between ovarian and colorectal cancer. In the uterus, adenocarcinomas that arise in the endocervix express greater amount of CEA than adenocarcinomas of the endometrial. This is reflected in the reported frequency of elevated plasma CEA levels : 68% in cervical cancer, and 34%

in endometrial cancer[40]. Squamous cell cancer, which represent 85% of the cervical cancer, also express CEA, but at more modest level. In a study on 205 patients, only 28% had plasma level above 5ng/ml. High levels indicated advance disease or lymph node metastases[41].

1.4.2 Genomic Markers

By cytogenetic examination, using a chromosome spread technique or cell flow cytometry, general genetic alteration have been identifying. Aneuploidy is a common finding in endometrial cancer and ovarian cancer[42][43]. There is a correlation between DNA ploidy abnormalities and grade of differentiation (more common in moderately and poorly differentiated lesions). Trisomy of chromosomes 1,7 and 10 and allelic loss at loci on chromosomes 3p (71%), 9q(38%) 10q(35%) and 17p(35%) have also reported in endometrial cancer[44]. Most ovarian and endometrial cancers over express of macrophage colony stimulating factor (M-CSF) and c-fms which encode the M-CSF receptor[45][46]. The macrophages secrete cytokines (tumor necrosis factor α and interleukins 1 and 6) that stimulate the growth of tumors[47]. Epidermal growth factor (EGF) and polo-like kinase (PLK) protein (contribute to regulation of the cell cycle) have been found to be expressed in most ovarian tumor, while the suppressor gene p53 defective[9][48]. However, the clinical significance of these genomic markers has not yet been established.

1.4.3 Enzymatic Markers

Lactate dehydrogenase (LDH) and heat stable alkaline phosphatase (HSAP) have been also considered as potential tumor markers in gynecology cancers.

The glycolytic enzyme LDH aroused a considerable interest in oncology since Warburg[49] reported increased rate of glucose utilization producing more lactate by tumor cells. LDH is often elevated in epithelial ovarian cancer[50], as in many solid malignancies[51], making it a non-specific tumor markers. In germ cell tumor, the two isoenzymes (LDH-1 and LDH-2) are increased and their activity appear to parallel the response to therapy [52]. Serum LDH levels were documented to be elevated in cervical cancer even at the early stage of the disease and in combination with other biomarker was more beneficial for diagnosis and treatment monitoring of patients[53][54].

Alkaline phosphates (ALP) was one of the first examples of tumor associated enzymes[55]. The heat stable alkaline phosphatase (HSAP, Regan isoenzyme) has been found in a variety of solid tumors and in 6-64% of ovarian cancer patients[56][57]. The marker level did not correlated to tumor burden or prognosis and half of the patients lost the marker during progression.

1.4.4 Hormonal Markers

Gonadotropin hormones (LH, FSH) can function as tumor markers in gonadal stromal tumor in addition to estrogen and androgen[17]. Inhibins, which are produced in ovarian granulosa cells, cause a specific suppression of pituitary FSH release. Radioimmunometric determination of inhibin has proven to be reliable marker in the monitoring of granulosa cell tumors[58].

1.4..4.1 Human Chorionic Gonadotropin (hCG)

Since the discovery of human chorionic gonadotropin (choriogonadotropin) hormone by Hirose[59] and Ascheim and Zondek[60], its measurement has been the basis of pregnancy diagnosis and, a marker for many trophoblastic and nontrophoblastic tumors.

This hormone is synthesized by the trophoblastic cells of the placenta during the early weeks of pregnancy. Human chorionic gonadotropin stimulates the ovarian corpus luteum to produce progesterone until the placenta it self acquires the ability to produce this pregnancy sustaining steroid[61]. An increasing evidence supports the synthesis of hCG in small quantities by the pituitary[62].

Human chorionic gonadotropin belongs to the glycoprotein hormones family (also includes hLH, hTSH, hFSH) whose members share a common α-subunit (contains

92 amino acids) and vary in their β-subunit. Each subunit is produced by a separate gene, the α subunit is encoded by a single gene present on chromosome 6q21.1-q23 whereas cluster of seven nonallelic genes located on chromosome 19q13.3 encoded for β-subunit of hCG(hCGβ). (One or more of these genes may preferentially expressed during pregnancy and tumor genesis)[63][64]. The β-subunit confer biological specificity; in humans, hCGβ and hLHβ are closly related subunits with 82% identity, and this reflects a common biological function for these two hormones.The hCGβ (contains 145 amino acids) further differs from that of hLHβ (contains 114 amino acids) by the 24-amino acid carboxy terminal polypeptide extension (CTP). It has been suggested that this glycosylated extension may impart extra solubility and in vivo circulation life time to hCG[65)].

Human chorionic gonadotropin could be purified from pregnancy urine by a combination of organic precipitation, ion exchange chromotography, and gel filtration[66].

A- Chemical Structure of hCG

The primary structure of α and β subunits for hCG were determined in 1973[67][68]. There are five disulfide bridges in the α-subunit and six in the β-subunit (these are conserved across the family). Human chorionic gonadotropin (38,633 Dalton) is approximately 30% carbohydrate by weight and contains both complex biantennary N-asparagine linked and simple O-serine linked. Each carbohydrate moiety terminates in sialic acid, but considerable carbohydrate heterogeneity result in a wide isoelectric point (pI) distribution of the hormone (pI generally 3-6 and as high as 10 for asialo forms of the hormone). The hCG produced in trophoblaste disease exhibits greater carbohydrate heterogeneity (such as triantennary structures) and some cancers produce only asialo hCG[66]. Removal of the terminal sialic acid residues markedly reduce the half-life of hormone in the circulation by enhancing binding to hepatocyte lectin and thus clearance from the blood stream. The carbohydrate moieties of hCG also played a role in hormone secretion, stability, folding and subunit assembly[99]. In vitro, studies with deglycosylated hormone generally indicate a greater loss of biological response than receptor binding. It is believed that the carbohydrate chains bind to a lectin-like membrane component to give the biological response. It was further found that the carbohydrate in the α-subunit was more important in the hormone function than that present in the β-subunit, which seems to be important to maintain the proper conformation of the hormone[70][71].

Various attempts have been made to construct three dimensional (3D) model of hCG[72-78]. Based on amino acid sequence and information; accumulated from chemical modifications (oxidization, deglycossylation, desialyation, reduction), enzymatic modifications (nicks, fragmentation and deletion of fragments), cross reactions, disulfide pairings, molecular biology studies (site directed mutagenesis, chimeric hormone constructs) with monoclonal antibodies(MAb) mapping of surface epitopes, spectral analyses (especially circular dichroism (CD)) and diffraction analyses (X-ray diffraction of hydrogen floride-hCG crystals), multi wavelength anomalous diffraction (MAD)); the proposed structure of hCG is predominantly composed of β structure with three helical segments, two in the α and one in the β-subunit. The antiparallel β- strands in each subunits are joined by three hairpin loops. Both subunits structure like some protein growth factors (NGF, TGF-β and PDGF-ββ) contain the so-called cysteine knot motif by three disulphide bonds (cys I-IV, cys II-V, cys III-VI). The heterodimer is stabilized by a segment of the β-subunit which wraps around the α-subunit and is covalently linked like a seat belt by cys 26-cys110. This hetrodimer has a large area of interface with only a small hydrophobic core. The overall topology of hCG subunit is shown in (Fig. 3).

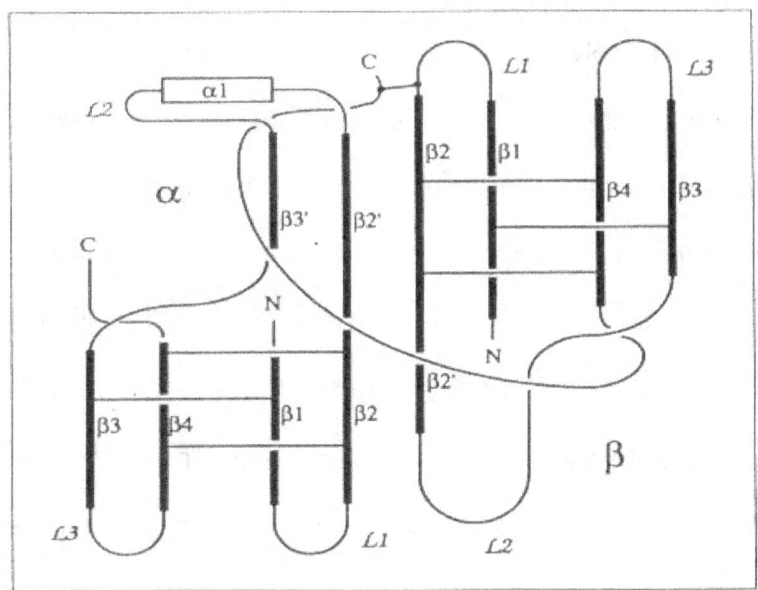

fig.3 A schematic drawing of the hCG dimer topology

B- Molecular Forms of hCG

Various molecular forms of hCG (intact or modified), free subunits (intact or modified), and degradation products are present in biologic fluid, tissues of normal and tumoral organs and reference preparations[79].

Intact hCG is defined as heterodimer comprising the two mature α and β subunits. Its levels in the sera of normal nonpregnant women increase with age, and higher than in men[80][81]. In women <50 year the upper reference limit is 8.6 pmol/l (2.9 Iu/L), and in those >50 years is 15-5 pmol/L (5.3 Iu/L), where the level of hCG in urine is < 2 pmol/mmol creatinine. In contrast, hCG levels are 2-6 pmol/L (0.7-2.1 Iu/L) in sera of healthy men. Plasma intact hCG rises exponentially during the first trimester of pregnancy, reaching a peak of 25-30 µg/ml at 8-10 weeks. Following a rapid decreases until 15 weeks, a slower but continuous fall is observed up to delivery. Interestingly, amniotic hCG levels are <20% of maternal serum level at all times of gestation[79].

Free hCGβ refers to the non-combined β-subunit consisting of a glycosylated 23KD single chain polypeptide. This form appears to be devoid of any biologic role during pregnancy (the peak level reaches 50-70 ng/ml between 8-10 week)[79]. In normal individuals, free hCGβ serum values are extremely low (never excceding 4.5 pmol/L) while this form is most often secreted in nontrophoblastic tumors[82].

Free hCGα refers to non combined α-subunit. Although it appears to have a structure identical to that of the combined α subunit of hCG, its carbohydrate composition is quite different which prevents combination[83]. This form may have a biologic role in pregnancy independent form that of hCG, where its level in serum slowly increase up to 18 weeks to reach a peak of 30-50ng/ml. In healthy individuals, levels up to 3000 pg/ml are present in sera originate in the pituitary gland[62]. Free hCGα may increase in pituitray tumors.

Beta -Core Fragment of hCGβ (hCGβcf), is small forms (10KD) immunoreactivity identify. Its two disulfide-bridged peptides lacking the amino acid sequences 1-5, 41-54 and 93-145 and corbohydrate structure changes of hCGβ[84]. It has been demonstrated that HCGβcf is primarily product of renal degradation of hCGβ, although some fragments may originate from either placenta or cleavage in the circulation. hCGβcf is the most abundant fragment of hCGβ in pregnancy urine and is also found in the urine of patients with a broad spectrum of malignancies and benign tumors. Circulating hCGβcf is almost undetectable, while levels of 0.51-1.25 pmol/mmol creatinine are found in urine of healthy women[69]

Nicked hCG (hCGn or hCGβn), are detectable in a significant proportion of both hCG and its free β subunit of normal and tumoral origins, as a result of intrachain proteolysis nicking within the β44-49 region [85][86]. The hCG appears to be uns Table and rapidly dissociates and weakly recognized by MAb. Furthermore, some results indicate that hCGβn is an intermediary form in the metabolism of hCG, and further cleavage to hCGβcf.

Several other molecules are detectable mostly in tumors, due to the modification of peptide structures both in hCGα and hCGβ such as N-terminal heterogeneity hCGα, mutant hCGα, large hCGα and CTP, hyperglycosylated hCG[87].

C- Production and Metabolism of hCG

Both normal placental cells as well as neoplastic trophoblastic cells, and sperm cells in the male synthesize and secrete hCG and its free subunits[88]. Human chorionic gonadotropin plays a critical role in the maintenance of the corpus luteum during the first 4 to 6 week of gestation to produce progesterone to keep the endometrial intact where the blastocyst is implanted, hCG also stimulates the testosterone production by the developing tests in males Fetuses[79]. The physiological processes regulating hCG production are not well understood. It is likely that its biosynthesis is dependent on the stage of differentiation of the trophoblastic cells and regulated by several autocrine and paracrine factors acting through cellular signals on the regulatory elements of the α- and β-subunit genes[89].

About 80% of hCG is metabolized in liver and renal tissue and excreted predominately as hCGβcf, whereas 20% of circulated hCG is excreted unmodified. In normal individuals, the plasma half-life of hCG is about 24-36 hours. Its clearance includes an initial, fast component ($t_{1/2}$ of 5-6h) and a second, slower component ($t_{1/2}$ of over 24 h)[69].

D- Clinical Use of hCG Determinations

Diagnosis of Pregnancy and Related Disorders: Immunochemical determination of hCG in serum or more commonly in urine, is the main method for diagnosis of pregnancy. In serum a discrimination limit of 10 Iu/L is often used [79].

Spontaneous abortion is the most common complication of pregnancy, and abnormally low serum hCG concentrations are often observed in these patients.

Serial determinations of hCG in serum in combination with sonography are much used for diagnosis this condition [66].

Decreasing or slowly increasing hCG concentration during early pregnancy may also indicate ectopic pregnancy (implantation of the blastocyst outside the uterus)[66].

The potential usefulness of either hCG or its free subunits(in combination with AFP) in prenatal screening for chromosomal abnormalities (particularly Down's syndrome), was the subject of intense debate[90][91]. While the mean hCGβ value in cases of trisomy 21 is significantly higher than in unaffected cases, the median value in trisomy 18 was found to be significantly lower.

Placental and Testicular Trophoblastic Tumors: Infact hCG and free hCGβ are ideal tumor marker for gestational trophoblastic disease (GTD ʷchoriocarcinoma,and hydatidiform mole[92]ʷ)and testicular germ cell tumors[93].The ratio of hCGβ to intact hCG is higher in patients with malignant than with benign trophoblastic tumors, which used for diagnosis. Measurement of blood intact hCG can be utilized for the therapeutic monitoring of GTD. Molecular heterogeneity has been demonstrated in the carbohydrate structure of hCG in choriocarcinoma, hCG is substantially diminished in sialic acid content and is composed of tri and tetra-antennary carbohydrate moieties[94].

Human chorionic gonadotropin or its free subunits presents in (80%) of sera patients with nonseminomatous testicular tumors, where hCG is elevated to more than 20,000 pg/ml[93]. Indeed, hCG, free hCG, AFP are the Most useful markers for the diagnosis, prognosis, and follow up of these malignancies[95]. Measurement of hCG in CSF is done when cerebral metastasis are suspected (ratios of hCG in CSF to hCG in serum exceed 1:60). In seminoma testicular cancer, hCG is elevated in 16% of patients[96].

Nontrophoblastic Tumors : The presence of hCG and its subunits in the tumor itself or in the serum and malignant effusions of patients with nontrophoblastic and nongonadal tumors were investigated. Numerous investigators, using immunochemical procedures, have demonstrated that cancers of the breast, uterus, lung, ovary, cervix, gastrointestinal tract, bladder, liver produce elevated concentrations of hCG or its subunits.

a-*Blood studies:* Early results employing radioimmuno assay(RIA) for hCG indicated that a great variety of malignant tumors expressed hCG[97-102]. The overall incidence was in the range of 19%-30% of all tumors studied. The levels of hCG were only moderately increased and shown variable correlation to tumor stage, histological grading or clinical course. Therefore, the clinical value of determine hCG in serum for diagnosing and monitoring patients with non-trophoblastic malignancies remains controversial. Studies with highly specific sandwich procedures and effective MAb showed that free hCGβ is mainly elevated while intact hCG and hCGα are slightly elevated or within the normal range in the sera of nontrophoblastic cancers. The malignancies that exhibited the greatest incidence are gynecologic cancers, tumor of the head, neck, lung, gastrointestinal tract tumors, and melanoma[102-111]. These studies suggested that free hCGβ is highly diagnostic of malignancy in general and defines a subgroup of aggressive nongonadal malignancies.

b-*Urine studies:* hCGβcf, free hCGβ, and asialo hCG have been reported in urine of different malignancies employing two soild phase capture antibodies[112][104][105]. Using a cutoff of 0.2ng/ml for hCGβcf, 59% of the cervical and endometrial and 70% of the ovarian cancers patients exceeded this level[113]. It has been suggested that the hCGβcf in the urine of patients is due to the degradation of the free hCGβ produced by these cancers.

c-*Effusion fluids studies:* Free hCGβ immunoreactive material has been reported in ascetic and tumor cyst fluids of patients with non trophoblastic cancers (including gynecologic cancers) more than intact hormone[106][107]. Free hCGβ levels have shown to be higher in malignant ascites as compared to the corresponding plasma values of the same patients. Determining free hCGβ in malignant effusions enhanced the sensitivity of this marker as compared to serum.

d-Tissues studies: Human chorionic gonadotropin in the cell is present in two pools, a secretary pool and membrane pool. The latter becomes an intrinsic part on determination hCG on the cancer cell surface. Various investigations on cultured cancer cells (including cells form nasopharynx, lung, cervix, bladder, breast, endometrial, colon, prostate, oral cancers, leukemia's, lymphomas, and retinoblastomas), using flow cytomatry technique, demonstrated the expression of membrane associated hCG and its subunit[114-124]. These studies showed high expression of free hCGβ than intact hCG and there was no relationship between the hCGβ positivity and the histological type or morphological features of tumor, but a number of authors have suggested that tumor which expresses hCG will pursue amore aggressive course and has a worse prognosis[125]. Analyses also done on extracted of media of cultured caner cells, reflecting the secretary pool or total cell pools. Other techniques such as immunohistochemical techniques were used to identify hCG in tumor and normal tissues[126-137]. Positive staining for hCG were found in, ovarian, cervical, colorectal, gastric, hepatoblastoma, large bowel, urothelial and breast cancers tissue. Authors also reported the stimulation of the growth of several tumor cell lines by hCG[138-141]. These findings with other results which confirmed that hCG has also chemical and physiologic properties of growth factor[76][77], have provided a scientific basis for studies of, prevention from, and control of the cancer by active or passive immunization against hCG and its subunits[142]. Some studies used anti hCG vaccines which originally was developed for fertility control[143][144]. In addition to that, studies on cluster of genes encoding the hCGβ demonstrated that five nonallelic genes are transcribed in vivo with highly variable level of expression in first trimester placenta tissue, whereas normal nontrophoblastic tissue express 2 allelic hCGβ genes. In tumor tissue collected from patient with breast bladder, prostate, thyroid cancer found that up to 61% of these tumors expressed four nonallelic hCGβ genes different from that of normal tissue.

These findings provide the basis for a simple test that may be useful for the molecular diagnosis of nontrophsblastic cancer[64][115].

E- Determination Methods of hCG

Immunological methods are nearly exclusively used for clinical determination of hCG[82], while assessment of the potency of hCG preparations to be used for pharmaceutical purposes should be performed by bioassays.

Biological Methods

a-<u>In vivo methods</u>: These bioassays measure the response of gonadal tissue to hCG in various animals (mice, rabbits, frogs). These methods are no longer widely used because its susceptible to yielding spurious results due to variation in the metabolic clearance rates of the forms of hCG being assessed and are based on animal – derived rather than Human chorionic gonadotropin receptor[69].

b-<u>In vitro methods</u>: Two methods have been widly used for assessing the hLH-like bioactivity of hCG, one is based on the rat interstitial cell testosterone response (RICT assay)[145] and the other on the mouse interstitial cell response (MICT assay)[146]. These methods have the advantage of the low detection limit but the limitation is their lack of specificity (hLH activity, factors modulate cellular responses) and heterologous nature of the systems. Homologous bioassays have been constructed with the modern techniques of molecular biology, where the human hCG receptor gene has been cloned and transfected into cells to produce human receptors[147].

Binding Methods

Binding assay can utilize antibodies or receptor as binding protein.

a. <u>Competitive Immunoprocedures</u>

Radioimmuno assay(RIA), and Receptor methods: Pregnancy test is the first specific immunoprocedueres (qualitative agglutination inhibition methods) in which, latex particles or sheep red blood cell coated with the hCG, mix with the urine sample and then with a solution containing antibodies to the hCG. Presence of hCG in urine inhibits agglutination. This method is still widely utilized, especially as in-house methods[69].

The quantitative specific immunoprocedures for hCG were typical competitive immunoprocedure in which the radio active iodine ^{125}I-hCG competes with sample analyze for binding to anti-hCG. Increased hCG in sample, decreased bound radio activity. These methods are still used widely for measurement of serum and urine hCG levels[148][69].

Another type of assays systems available for serum hCG determination is a radioreceptor assay (RRA). This method is based on the competition between the hCG in the serum and a ^{125}I-hCG for binding to hCG receptor present in tissue [69].

b. <u>Non – competitive immunoprocedures</u>:

Non competitive immunometric with labeled antibody (sandwich or two-site immunometric methods) are quantitative methods for hCG and its subunits with low detection limit, large measurement range. The labeled anti hCG reacts with sample hCG bound to solid phase anti hCG. Diffferent labels are used such as enzyme, fluorescent, and luminescent. The specificity of sandwich methods is defined by the reactivity and recognition ability of the antibodies (β •→ α, β •→ β, αβ •→ β, βcf •→ β, βCTP •→ α, α •→ α) where •-- capture antibody and → tracer antibody[79](Fig.4).

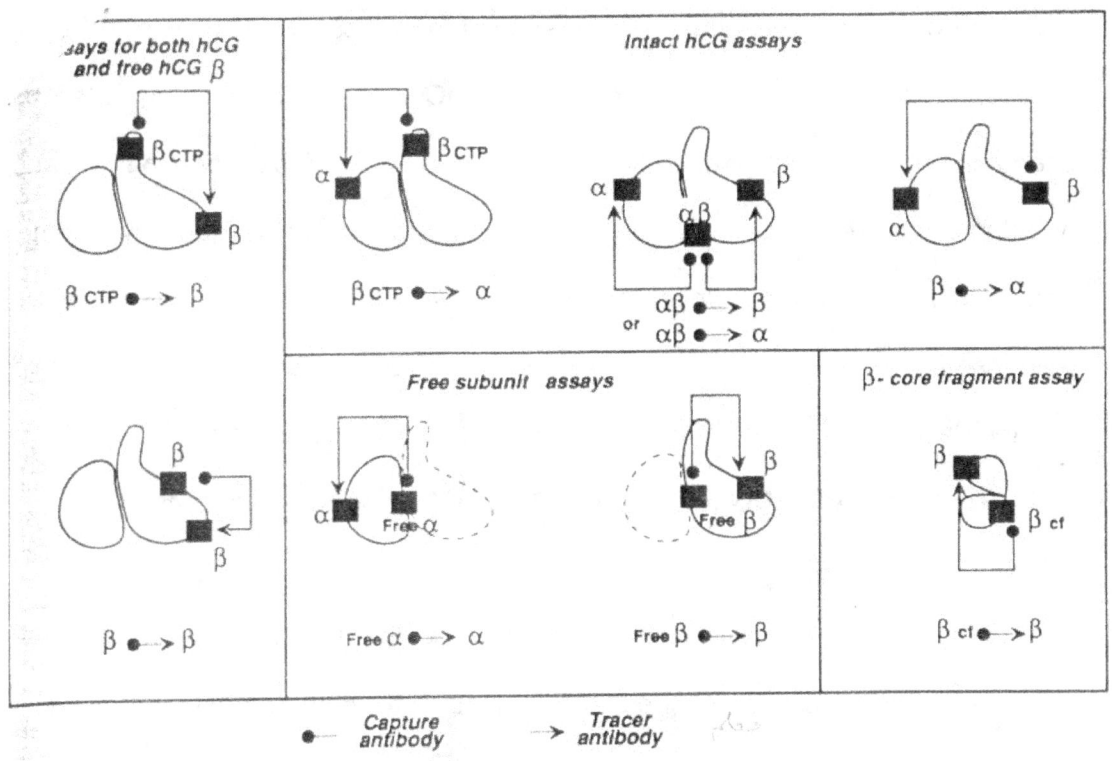

Fig.4 Schematic representation of the sandwich methods used for the measurement of hCG, its free subunits, or hCGcf[79]

1.5 Human Chorionic Gonadotropin Receptor (hCG-R)

Human chorionic gonadotropin receptor is a cell surface protein, present on testicular leydig cells and on ovarian theca, interstitial, luteal, and mature granulosa cells. In both males and females, the hCG-R recognizes the pituitary hormone LH. In the pregnant female, the same receptor also recognizes hCG[149].

The hCG-R belongs to a subfamily of glycoprotein hormone receptor within the G protien-coupled receptor family (whose members are characterized by the common structural feature of seven transmembrance domains)[150].

Although there are differences in the response duration, affinity and dissociation rate of hCG for the hCG-R as compared to LH, it is generally believed that both hormones bind to and activate the receptor similarity. Studies to date indicate that the cAMP second messenger system is the predominant pathway stimulated by either LH or hCG. Yet, it has been reported that stimulation with LH or hCG leads to activation of phospholipase C, resulting in formation of inositol phosphates and elevation in intracellular Ca^{2+} $[Ca^{2+}]$[151][152]. The responsiveness of a given target cell to hCG or LH can be modulated by alteration in the number of cell surface receptor such as homologous and hetrologous down regulation, as a results of internalization and lysosomal degradation of hormone- receptor complex[149]. Desensitization (reduction in response intensity) has also been observed for hCG-R it has been hypothesized that the desentization occurs as a result of receptor phosphorylation[153].

1.5.1 Structure of the hCG-R and the Nature of Hormone –Receptor Interaction

Structural studies have been hampered by the low abundance of hCG receptor, nonetheless, researchers have made sufficient progress in this area. Data from chemical crosslinking of labed hCG to the receptor, immunoprcipitation of a biosynthetically labeled hCG-R, purification of the receptor, have led to the estimation of the overall size and structure of this receptor[154-158]. Studies on the cDNA and genomic clones for hCG-R have yielded more detailed information on the structure and function[147][159-161]. The antibodies developed to the receptor have confirmed the topology of this receptor and are being used to address structure function relationship[149][154]. All these studies established that hCG-R is a single chain glucoprotien of 85-93 KDa. Its composed of two halves of equal size., the N-terminal extracellular hydrophilic, exodomain of ~ 350 amino acid residues and the membrane associated intracellular C-terminal endodomain of ~334 amino acids residues, which includes seven hydrophobic transmembrane helices and three cytoplasmic loops with three extracellular loops that link the seven transmembrane domains (Fig.5) The hCG-R is encoded by 11 exons located on chromosome 2 p21, the first 10 of which code for the exodomain and the 11th for the endodomain.

hCG Receptor

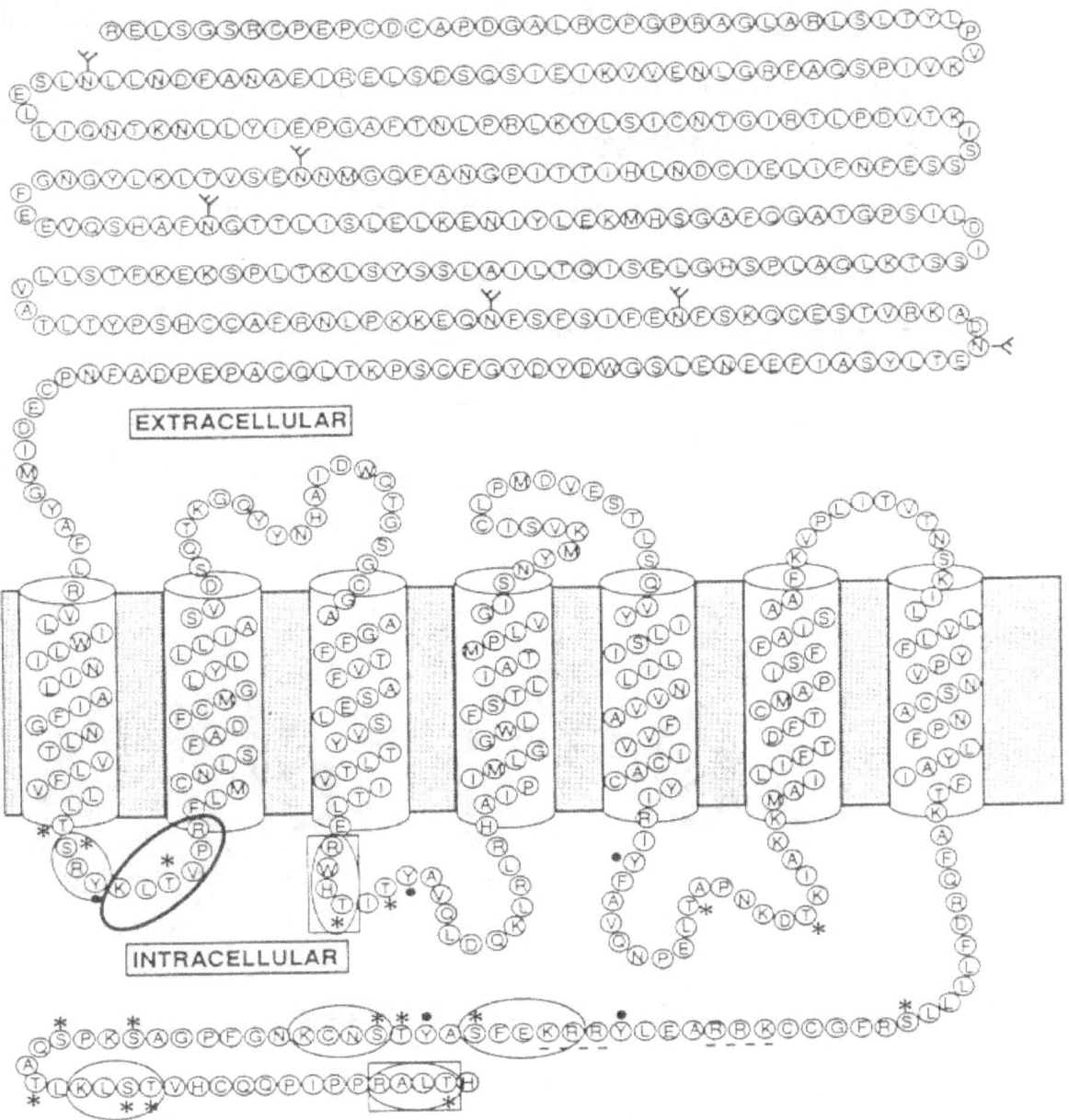

Fig.5 Amino acid sequence, orientation, and proposed topology of the hCG receptor in the plasma membrane. Potential sites for N-linked glycosylation are shown by the branch-like structures. The sequences underlined with dashes in the cytoplasmic tail mark two clusters of basic amino acids which might represent potential tryptic cleavage sites. Potential intracellular sites for phosphorylation and denoted by asterisks (serine and threonine residues) or dark dots (tyrosine). The rectangles denote weak consensus sequences for cAMP-dependent protein kinase –catalyzed phosphorylation. The ovals and heavy ovals denotes weak and strong consensus sequences for c kinase-catalyzed phosphorylation[154].

Results from mutational analysis[162-164], chimeric construction[165], synthetic peptide studies[166] and chemical modification of the receptor[154] showed that the hormone binding and activation processes are separable. The large extacellular domain of hCG with six sites for N-linked glycosylation and (8-9) leucine –rich repeats (LRR) is responsible for high selectivity and affinity hormone binding without hormone action[167-170]. LRR are thought to form a crescent with concave inner surface consisting of β sheets which may bind hormone (Fig.6)

Hormone Contact Site of LH/CG Receptor

Fig.6 Schematic model for the interaction of the hCG receptor exodomain with hCG. Hormone interacts with the inner face of the crescent structure of the receptor[173].

Activation, in contrast, has been identified with transmembrance domain [171]. The molecular mechanism involves the initial high affinity contact of hCG with receptor exodomain, then the resulting complex (may not be thermodynamically stable) undergoes conformational changes and makes secondary low affinity interactions with exoloops of membrane associated domain(Fig.7), causing an allosteric structural change in the endodomain which leads to signal generation and hormone action[172][150].

Fig.7 Schematic presentation of the receptor-hCG interaction. hCG bind to the N-terminal segment of the receptor and the hCG-N-terminal segment interacts with exo loops to generate a signal[150].

The initial high affinity interaction includes multiple contacts between the exdomain and both subunits of the hormone[173][174]. The precise hormone contact sites in the exodomain are unclear. The most putative contact sites are αC-terminal region, N-oligosaccharide at αAsn^{52}, and unique αhelix in the α-subunit, as well as unusual loop (seat belt) in the β-subunit and the peripheral β-hair pin loop of both subunits[175]. Between the initial interaction and the signal generation, hCG and receptor undergo conformational changes. Studies including photochemical crosslinking of hCG, mutational analysis of the receptor and serial truncation has been demonstrated a structural changes of hCG involving the intersubunit interaction[162][164][176-177].

1.5.2 The Role of hCC-R in Nongonadal Tissues and Tumor Tissues

It has long believed that the hCG-Rs were present only in gonads. But the studies, using immunocytochemistry method and MAb for receptor or reverse transcription polymerase chain reaction technique, have demonstrated that various female as well as male nongonadal tissues (uterus, placenta, fetal membrane, deciduas, fallopian tubes, brain, breast, skin) contain low levels of hCG-R protein and hCG-R transcripts (cancer tissues are among these tissues)[178-187]. Moreover the direct action of ectopically synthesis hCG in regulating the growth of various cell types and its role in various cancers, implies the existence of the corresponding receptors in these tissues.

Studies on nonpregnant human uteri, demonstrated not only the presence but also different cellular distribution of hCG-R, where epithelial cells contain more receptors than that stromal cells of endometrial in turn, contain more than myometrial and vascular smooth muscle[178][188]. The hCG-R are increased from the proliferation to the secretary phase of the cycle. These differences suggest that other hormones regulate the receptor, which regulated different functions. Evidences from in vitro studies supported these suggestion, for example , hCG was reported to have a relaxing effect on porcine myometrium[189] and can increase cAMP levels and progesterone synthesis in rat uterus[190]. The expression of receptor mRNA had been found higher in myometrial then in human endometrial blood vessels ,and there is possibility that hCG could an directly increase uterine blood flow [187]. Human chorionic gonadotropin may regulate epithelial cell by increasing the local synthesis of steroid hormones[190]. In vitro , hCG can directly regulate proliferation of human myometrial smooth muscle cells causing hyperplasia as well as hypertrophy[188]. Increasing expression of receptor gene in human endometrial cancer has also been obtained [184].

Studies on human placenta, fetal membranes, decidua have been shown the presence of receptors as well as cellular localization differences and changes from mid to term pregnancy suggesting that hCG may regulate their function. In fact, there are data from in vitro studies support this possibility, in placenta, high hCG-R concentration have been shown to increase cAMP formation[191], glycogen breakdown[192], aromatization of androgens to estrogens[193], and interconversion of estron to estradiol[194]. In decidua, high hCG concentration have been shown to directly stimulate prolactin synthesis, which in turn, has been inhibited placental hCG synthsis. This finding indicates the presence of hCG- influenced short loop positive and negative regulatory mechanisms within the human fetoplacental unit[195][196]. Investigation for the presence of functional hCG-R in human breast, revealed that normal epithelial cell, benign lesion, and cancer biopsies content hCG-R[183][197]. The intensity of the immunolabeling of hCG-R varied in individual biopsies. The presence of receptor mRNA was also confirmed. In the breast, it has been proposed that hCG provokes differenentiation, which in turn renders the cells less susceptible to neoplastic transformation[198]. This mechanism would explain the decreased occurrence of breast cancer in women who had on early pregnancy. Studies on human breast cell lines showed the functional presence of hCG-R that can bind hCG to exert a direct antiproliferative effect on human breast epithelial cells through secretion of inhibin and decreasing estrogen receptor[199]. Indeed hCG has been shown to exert either stimulatory or inhibitory effects on the growth of various cancer in vitro. In bladder, lung and endometrial cancer as well as choriocarcinoma, hCG and/or its subunits promote the growth of these cancers while in breast and prostate cancers are growth inhibiting[115].

The Aim of the Work

The aim of this work includes the following :

1-Investigation the presence of intact hCG and free hCGβ in sera and tissues of patients with endometrial and epithelial ovarian cancers.

2-Development a quantitative radiorecptor assay for detection and analysis of membrane-associated hCG-Rs of human cancer tissues of endometrial and epithelial ovarian cancers.

3-Purification and characterization the hCG-Rs of epithelial ovarian cancer from detergent soluble membrane extracts .

4-Determination of the kinetic parameters of the binding reaction of hCG with it's receptor in epithelial ovarian cancer.

5-Investigation the CEA in the sera and tissues of endometrial and epithelial ovarian cancers patients.

6-Evaluation the levels of LDH, and ALP enzymes activities in sera of endometrial and epithelial ovarian cancers patients and analysis the different isoenzymes and forms of them.

7-Measuring the concentration of Copper, Zinc, and Calcium elements in sera of patients with endometrial and epithelial ovarian cancers.

Chapter Two

Human Chorionic Gonadotropin in Sera and Tissues of Patients with Gynecologic Cancers

Human Chorionic Gonadotropin in Sera and Tissues of Patients with Gynecologic Cancers

Abstract

In the present study, the presence of intact hCG and free hCGβ in sera and tissues of patients with gynecologic cancers was investigated by radioimmunoassy for these two forms of hCG. Intact hCG and free hCGβ level was found to be elevated above the reference value(>5mIU/ml) in the sera of 7 out of 14 patients (50%) with epithelial ovarian cancer and 4 out of 9 (44%) patients with endometrial cancer. There was no significant difference between the mean age of hCG positive and hCG negative cancer patients, but hCG-positive patients were significantly older in the benign group. The intact hCG and free hCGβ in malignant conditions (87.6 ± 47.9mIU/ml) were higher than in benign conditions (11.2 ± 2.2mIU/ml) ($P< 0.05$).Circulating intact hCG and free hCGβ could be demonstrated in early as well as in advanced stage of gynecologic cancers. After radical surgery,4 out of 6 hCG-positive patients turned to be normal, and 2 of them remained positive.

In malignant tissue extracts, the intact hCG and free hCGβ were significantly higher than in the corresponding sera samples of benign tumor samples. Elevation intact hCG and free hCGβ in tissues(>5 mIU/ml) was found in 100% of patients with gynecologic cancers. The level of intact hCG and free hCGβ exceeded 10mIU/ml in all of 23 malignant tissue samples whereas not exceeded 10mIU/ml in all of 25 benign tissue samples. In this respects, measurement of hCG in tumor tissue may be of higher diagnostic value as serum measurement.

Introduction

Human chorionic gonadotropin is a clinically relevant marker of trophoblastic and nontrophoblastic cancers. Most studies have focused on serum determination of hCG, which have been reported to be elevated in a significant portion of patients with various nontrophoblastic cancers including gynecologic cancers [97-111]. The elevation of hCG reported vary considerably for similar cancer. This is possibly due to differences in patient selection and assay characteristic. Recently, the utilization of monoclonal antibodies, highly specific for intact hCG or its subunits have been re-evaluated the presence of hCG in the sera of nontrophoblastic tumors[102-111]. Several studies have shown that either hCG or its subunits may be localized to a variety of nontrophoblastic tissues and was extrac Table from malignant and normal human tissues[126-137]. Expression of membrane-associated hCG was found to be a phenotypic marker characteristic of all evaluated cultured human cancer cell lines, irrespective to their type or origin [114-125]. A stimulation of the growth of several tumor cells by hCG had also been reported[138-141].

In present work, a re-evaluation of presence of intact hCGand free hCGß in sera samples of patients with endometrial and epithelial ovarian cancer was carried out using a highly sensitive and specific radioimmunoassay (RIA) for these forms of hCG. Determination of intact hCG and free hCGß in these malignant tissues had been carried out to further definition of the role of hCG as tumor marker,

Materials and Methods:

2.1 Chemicals

All laboratory chemicals and reagents were of analar grade. PMSF (phenyl methyl salfonyl flouride),Tris (hydroxymethylaminaomethane), Glycerol, HCL, EDTA, and BSA were obtained from Fluka. NaOH, Na_2CO_3, $CuSO_4$, $MgCl_2$ and Folin reagent were obtained from BDH.

Intact hCG and free hCGß ^{125}I RIA kit was provided by Diasorin which contain one vial of ^{125}I-hCG tracer (I µg/ml); one vial of rat-monoclonal hCGß antibody recognizes hCGß within holo-hCG as well as in its free form; one vail of precipitating goat anti-mouse serum (second antibody) in polymer solution, one vial of 90 mIU/ml hCG as control;one vial of hCG blank (0 mIU/ml); five vials of hCG standards with concentrations ranging of (5-200 mIU/ml); one vial of hCG calibrator at 50 mIU/ml.

2.2 Apparatus

The apparatus used during this study were, LKB gamma counter type 1270 Rack, cooling centrifuge type Hettich, LKB UV-Visible record spectrophtometers, Unicam pH meter, Memmert water bath, Memmert incubator, homogenizer type HO and SM shaker.

2.3 Patients

The study groups consisted of 82 women with gynecologic disease (age range between 22-80 years).Histological diagnosis was available in all cases. Malignant tumor was present in 23 patients (age range between 38-80), the tumor site was the endometrial adenocarcinoma in 9 and the epithelial ovary in 14 {(serous11), mucinous(3)}. Staging was performed according to the FIGO. The benign condition was present in 59 patients (age range between 22-67),this group consisted of adenomyosis (4 cases), fibromyoma (20 cases), endometriosis (3 cases), follicular cyst(10 cases), serous cystadenom tumors (9 cases), mucinous tumors(3 cases) polycystic (6 cases) and dermiod cyst (4 cases). Thirty healthy female between the age of 20-65 served as the control group, it was confirmed that the individuals were not suffering from any disease at time of the study and did not receive any medication.

All patients were admitted for treatment to aL-Yarmook Hospital, Saddam Medical City, Saddam Collage of Medicine, Al-Arabi Private Hospital.

2.4 Collection of Specimens and Preparation of Tissue Homogenates.

Serum: All blood samples were collected before treatment in all cases using venipuncture. Additional sample were obtained from 6 patients postoperatively while they were still in hospital. The samples were allowed to clot before separation by centrifugation at 1500xg for 15 min. The sera were subjected to RIA measurement.

Tissue: Tumor tissue specimens were obtained from patients during surgical operating. For comparison two term pregnancy placentas from spontaneous normal vaginal deliveries were used. The tissues were brought to the laboratory on crushed ice and washed extensively with ice-cold physiological saline to remove blood then stored frozen until analysis. The frozen tissues were weighted, minced finely then, homogenized in 50 mM Tris/HCL, pH 7.4 containing (0.25 M sucrose, 1mM $MgCL_2$, 5 mM EDTA, 1mM PMSF) with a ratio of 1:4 (w:v) by homogenizer at setting (2.5) using three 20s periods of homogenization. The homogenate was then filtered through a nylon mesh sieve in order to eliminate fibers and cell debris then centrifuged at 600xg for 15min at 4^0c to remove the nuclei. The pellet was again homogenized and centrifuged. The above supernatants were pooled and subjected to RIA measurement and protein determination.

2.5 Quantitative Measurement of Intact hCG and Free hCGß

Intact hCG anf free hCGß of sera and tissues samples were measured using highly sensitive and specific RIA Kit. The assay protocol was described in Table (2.1)

Table (2.1) Assay protocol of intact hCG and free hCGß

	Total count (tracer)	hCG Blank (0mIU/ml)	hCG Standards (mIU/ml)						hCG Control (mIU/ml)	Patient sample
			5	10	25	50	100	200	90	X
Tube number	T_1, T_2	B_0 1,2	3,4	5,6	7,8	9,10	11,12	13,14	15,16	17,18
Standards, control, blank patients samples (µL)		←------------------------ 200 µL ---→								
^{125}I-hCGß red tracer (µL)	←------------------------------- 100 µL ---→									
^{125}I-hCGß blue antibody		←------------------------ 100 µL ---→								
	1. vortex mixing, incubation for 1h at room temp., total count set aside until counting in gamma counter									
Precipitating antiserum		←-----------------------1ml--→								
	1. Incubation for 5 min at room temp. 2. Centrifugation at 40°C for 15 min at 1500xg 3. Decantation 4. Counting for radioactivity in a gamma counter for 1min									

Calculation:

1. The standard curve was drawn by plotting the CPM bound for hCG standards versus their concentration (Fig 2.1)
2. The samples values of intact hCG and free hCGβ were read directly from the curve. Patients samples with assay values greater than 200 mIU/ml must be diluted.

Estimation of Protein Contents:

Protein was measured by the method of Lowry et.al.,[200] using bovine serum albumin as standard.

Statistical Analysis: Results were expressed as mean ± S.E.M. Student's t - test and one way analysis of variance were used for statistical comparisons and P values of less than 0.05 were considered statistically significant.

Results and Discussion:

Preoperative Data:

Results of hCG determination depend largely on the selection of antibody and the type of technique used. In present study, re-evaluation of the presence of intact hCG and free hCGβ subunit immunoreactivity in serum of patients with ovarian and endometrial cancer, using RIA assay with the lower limit of sensitivity of (1.5 mIU/ml) and monoclonal antibody recognize these forms of hCG, had been done.

Immunoreative intact hCG and free hCGß, was elevated (> 5mIU/ml) in the sera of 11 out of 23 patients (48%) with gynecologic cancers (range 22.1 -166 mIU/ml) as shown in Table (2.2). Intact hCG and free hCGß was found to be above normal range in the sera of 4 out of 9 patients (44%) suffering from endometrial cancer range (22.1 -110.5 mIU/ml); mean ± S.E.M (64.5± 41.8 mIU/ml) (Table 2.3). In patients with ovarian cancer (n=14), elevated intact hCG and free hCGß serum values were found in 7 of 14 (50%) , range (37.3 -166 mIU/ml).

Intact hCG and free hCGß production occurred exclusively in patients with serous ovarian neoplasm (Table 2.3). Analysis of the data indicated no significant difference in the occurrence of hCG in patients with endometrial and ovarian cancer ($P > 0.05$, NS). Furthermore, elevations of intact hCG and free hCGß in the sera from patients with ovarian cancer (100.55± 45.32) were significantly higher than in the sera from patients with endometrial cancer (64.6±41.8).

The mean age of intact hCG and free hCGß positive group (61.5± 12.1) was similar to that of intact hCG and free hCGß negative group (60±11.3) of patients with endometrial and ovarian cancers (Table 2.2).

In benign condition positive findings were made in 7 of 59 cases (12%) including adenomyosis and myomas of the uterus, and various form of benign ovarian tumors (Table 2.3). The elevation level of intact hCG and free hCGß varied between (8.3-14.4) mIU/ml. The mean elevation (11.2± 2.2) mIU/ml was smaller than in the malignant group (87.6± 47.9)mIU/ml ($p<0.05$), the percentages of elevation intact hCG and free hCGß in benign and malignant conditions are shown in Fig 2.2. In the benign group hCG-positive patients were significantly older (60.6 ±5.8 years) than hCG- negative patients (44.2±8; $p<0.05$; Table 2.2).

Human chorionic gonadotropin is one of the earliest embryonic gene products appearing in ontogeny. The finding of circulating hCG in association with cancers has been regarded generally as another expression of embryonic antigens in cancer. It's place in fetal survival and placental development has been related to its role in the control of "pseudo malignancy" because trophoblastic cell has angiogenic and invasive properties[201]. Trophoblasts express oncogenes and proto-oncogene[202][203] and demonstrate cytokine expression[204] and resistance to immune rejection that we associate with malignancy.

The percentage of elevated of intact hCG and free hCGß was (48%) for patients with gynecologic cancer. This is comparable to that reported by Grossmann et.al.,[107] (37%) for gynecologic cancers based immunoradiometric design. Crawford et.

al.,[111] demonstrated the usefulness of free hCGβ and hCG$_{βcf}$ in assessing prognosis of primary cervical cancer. De-Bruijn et.al.,[109] studied the progressive vulvar cancer(n=104) and found elevated free hCGβ in 50% of patients and indicated that the synthesis of free hCGβ can be increased during progression. Ind et.al.,[108] investigated the elevated free hCGβ and other tumor markers in women with primary epithelial ovarian cancer. They found a correlation between markers levels and cancer stage. Elevated levels of intact hCG or free hCGβ were found also by other authors in different nontrophoblastic tumors in addition to gynecologic cancers,such as tumors of the head and neck, lung cancer ,gastrointestinal track tumors and melanoma . Hoermann et.al.,[106] found elevated level of free hCGβ in 55% of patients with (breast, pancreas, colon, stomach, ovary, cervix, bladder and hepatocellular cancer), whereas intact hCG was not elevated in all serum malignant samples. Marcillac et.al.,[103] detected elevated free hCGβ level in 47% of bladder, 32% of pancreatic and 30% of cervical cancer, they also found low elevation level of intact hCG in the same patients (1.3%). Alfthan et.al.,[104] observed elevated levels of serum free hCGβ in 72% of pancreatic cancer and 86% of biliary cancer. Iles and colleagues[105] demonstrated that the incidence of free hCGβ was approximately 30% in serum of patients with bladder cancer and 15 out of 36 patients with pancreatic adenocarcinoma had elevated plasma hCGβ[110]. In all these studies, the hCG assay sensitivity was increased for nontrophoblastic cancers by inclusion of free hCGβ subunit measurements.These studies indicated that most hCG-producing malignancies secret hCGβ in addition to the intact hCG molecule and free hCGβ subunit may even be the major form of hCG in nontrophoblatic cancers .This pattern of secretion contrasts with that observed in pregnant women who display a predominant secretion of intact hCG in large excess[79] .The result of an earlier studies based intact hCG determination confirm this observation where the values obtained are low. Donaldson et.al.,[99] in their assessment of markers of gynecologic cancers found low percentage (22%) of patients has total hCG serum level greater than 5 mIU/ml . Rutanen et. al.,[97]. also found an elevation of total serum hCG in only 18% of gynecologic cancers. In early studies[97-101], the overall incidence was in the range of 18-25% of all tumors studies.

Serum intact hCG and free hCGβ levels were elevated in 44% of patients with adenocarcinoma of the uterus and in 64% of patients with serous epithelial ovarian cancers. On considering whether the histological type of tumor or cells give any clue of its ability to secrete hCG, it is obvious, by the spectrum of histological appearance of hCG-producing tumors, that the morphological features of neoplastic are not necessarily linked to hormone producing. Donaldson et.al.,[99] among their analysis of ovarian and cervical tumors found elevated levels of hCG in selected cases of epithelial ovarian cancer (serous 27%, endometriod 100%, mucinous 0%, and Granulosa cell 0%) whereas small-cell, keratinizing, and nonkeratinizing types of squamous carcinomas had elevated levels in 13, 40 and 20% of cases respectively of cervical cancer, while none of the cervical adenocarcinoma had elevated levels of hCG. Mohabeer et.al.,[128] when examining ovarian epithelial tumors, found no relationship between the hCGβ positive and the histological type of tumors, or whether the tumor was of a benign, or malignant type (with no trophoblatic proliferation), nor even the histological grade of malignant tumors .Other authors such as Collins et.al.,.[132] demonstrated that hCGβ positive was found in adenocarcinoma of the uterine cervix in which the cells of tumor have some histological resemblance to trophoblastic cells. Rutanen et.al.,[97]. did not find bias in the distribution of hCG in patients with poorly and well–differentiated endometrial cancer, while Mc Manus et.al.,[100] have commented that hCG positive was most frequent in poorly differentiated anaplastic tumors. There are also nongestational and extragonadal tumors which both produce hCG and bear a striking resemblance to trophoblastic neoplasms such that many authors use the term "choriocarcinomatous" to describe them. Cases have been reported with either poorly differentiated transitional cell carcinoma of the bladder or adenocarcinoma of the urothelial, stomach colon, and uterus[129-132].

Low elevated intact hCG and free hCGβ were found in 12% of patients with nonmalignant gynecologic tumors, and women with positive intact hCG and free hCGβ were older than women with negative intact hCG and free hCGβ, using cut off level 5mIU/ml. If we take an important consideration that hCG excreted in healthy subjects[80] and there are direct evidence for production of the intact hCG by the pituitary gland[62] and its expression is related to the age[81], then the elevated intact hCG and free hCGβ in benign group could be explained. It is highly likely that the low level of intact hCG and free hCGβ (11.2±2.2) found in the sera of nonmalignant gynecological patients originates from the pituitary gland and not from the tumor. This level is significantly low in comparison with malignant group (87.6±47.9).

Theories to explain the production of ectopic proteins in general involve the possibility of derepression of genes that are expressed in fetal life, or the recruitment of uncommitted cells, or the occurrence of random mutation[132]. These hypotheses assume that hCG are not a normal features of later life, but the presence of very low levels of hCG in both tissues and body fluids during normal metabolism and tissue turnover has been documented[136][137][81][80]. The source of such hCG in healthy subjects is postulated to be the normal stem cells of replicating tissues. If hCG is synthesized in many normal sites, then the neoplastic cells because of their increased number would produce larger quantities of stem cell proteins compared to the quantities produced by normal cells.

Circulating intact hCG and free hCGß could be demonstrated in early as well as in advanced stage of the two kinds of gynecologic cancers (Table 2.4). Of the 9 patients with endometrial cancer, intact hCG and free hCGß elevated in 2 out of 6 and 2 out of 3 of the stage I and II, respectively . The highest intact hCG and free hCGß serum level (110 mIU/ml) was found in women with the stage II, however the analytical data indicated no significant differences in serum intact hCG and free hCGß concentration between two stages of endometrial cancer (p>0.05). In ovarian cancer, intact hCG and free hCGß was elevated in 2 out of 5 (40%) of stage I and 5 out of 9 (56%) of stages (II –III (Table 2.4). The highest level of intact hCG and free hCGß was found in patients with stage III (166 mIU/ml), but also no significant different in the serum intact hCG and free hCGß concentration found between different stages. It was found no correlation between the concentration of intact hCG and free hCGß and the spread of the tumor.

Although only a few cases could be examined, women with invasive endometrial and ovarian cancer as assessed by staging had the highest serum concentration of intact hCG and free hCGβ, but difference between stages was not statistically significant. These results confirm previous observation from other investigations, which characterize hCG as a key factor defining the metastasis phenotype specifically of nontrophoblasic malignancies. Grossmann et.al.,[107] obtained that the advanced disease of cervical cancer was associated with elevated intact hCG and free hCGβ serum values (4/13 (31%) of stage II and 11/27(41%) of stages III-IV) , also obtained that women with more aggressive endometrial cancers had higher serum concentrations of intact hCG and free hCGβ. Sheth et.al.,[101] using RIA techniques, found elevated levels of serum hCG in 41% patients with squamous carcinomas of cervix FIGO stages II-IV with an increasing frequency in the higher clinical grades. Marcillic et.al.,[103] found that the production of free hCGβ was associated with tumors of high prognosis such as cancers of the lung, pancreas, and liver. Walker[127] also noted a relation between the presence of hCG and metastases of breast cancer. Syrigos[110] and de-Bruijn[109] also indicated, that the patients with elevated serum hCGβ had a worse progressive tumor compared with the group of normal hCGβ in patients with vulvar and pancreatic cancer.

The sensitivity, specificity and predictive value of the intact hCG and free hCGß in the diagnosis of gynecologic cancers are shown in Table 2.5. When pre-treatment serum intact hCG and free hCGß levels were compared between patients with benign and those with malignant gynecologic tumors, they distinguished the malignant from benign tumor with a predictive value of (73% and 80%) in uterine corpus and ovarian tumor, respectively. In all healthy females sera, intact hCG and free hCGß activity was measurable. All females showed levels within the upper limit of normal range (5mIU/ml) (Table 2.2). In women older than 45 years the mean concentration (4.8 ± 0.5 mIU/ml) was significantly higher than that of the women younger than 45 year (3.8± 0.8 mIU/ml). It is noteworthy that hCG was present at low levels (<5 mIU/ml) in serum of many cancer patients as well as in healthy women's and patients with benign disease (Fig 2.3).

Postoperative Data:

Intact hCG and free hCGß levels were postoperatively measured in 6 hCG – positive cancer patients who had undergone radical surgery including hysterectomy and ovariectomy. The blood was obtained from them in the first postoperative week, while they were still in hospital. The data showed reversion of serum intact hCG and free hCGß levels in 4 patients, while 2 remained hCG–positive (Table 2.6). On the basis of clinical examination no tumor was demonstrated in any of the 4 hCG negative patients, while the 2 hCG- positive patients had a metastasis (stage III). One of these 2 women, multiple serum specimens were obtained from her during the period of different weeks. intact hCG and free hCGß concentration paralleled the clinical course of this patient (Fig.2.4).

In several cases elevated intact hCG and free hCGβ levels returned to normal level after operation, and that indicate the hormone has been produced by the tumor itself, but in two ovarian cancer cases with metastasis, intact hCG and free hCGβ levels remained elevated after operation which give an example of usefulness of hCG in the following of patients with ovarian cancer. Crossmann et.al.,[107] reported the importance of intact hCG and free hCGβ in following the ovarian cancer cases and commented that for the optimal management of gynecologic cancer, multiple markers measuring could be helpful. Marcillac et.al.,[103] and Alfthan et.al.,[104] have also reported that free hCGβ is promising marker in diagnosis and following the bladder and pancreatic cancer. Donaldson et.al.,[99] obtained that measuring hCG with other markers could help to follow up patients with gynecologic cancers.

Malignant and Non Malignant Tissues:

Intact hCG and free hCGß immunoreactivity has been determined in tumor tissues of the patients with endometrial and ovarian cancer (n=23), and in tumor tissues of patients with the benign tumor (n=25). For comparison, placenta intact hCG and free hCGß content has also been determined in 2 term pregnancy women. In malignant tissues, intact hCG and free hCGß levels ranged between (14.5 -212 mIU/ml; Table 2.7). Statistical analysis of differences between blood serum and tumor tissue intact hCG and free hCGß content in patient with malignancies has been performed. The elevation of tissue intact hCG and free hCGß level appeared to be statistically significant than in the corresponding serum samples ($P<0.05$). Remarkably, of these 12 women, which showed normal serum values (<5mIU/ml) (Fig 2.5).

In 25 non-malignant tissues, intact hCG and free hCGß levels ranged from (5.3 - 9.5 mIu/ml), mean 8.19 ± 1 mIU/ml which were significantly lower than in the specimen from women with ovarian and endometrial cancer ($P<0.05$) (Table 2.7). If the upper limit of normal range for tissue as 10 mIU/ml, then 23 out of 23 (100%) of the malignant tissue samples were considered pathological and 25 out of 25 (100%) of the benign were judged normal.Determination of hCG in placenta had been obtained for comparison. The term pregnancy placenta gives higher level of intact hCG and free hCGß, even more than cancer tissue (371 ± 11 mIU/ml) (Table 2.7).

Effort to improve the diagnosis efficiency in gynecologic tumors has been made by assessing intact hCG and free hCGß in tumor tissues. Malignant cells are assumed to be source of ectopic hormone production, however, the rate at which hCG is actually released into the circulation may vary considerably. Consequently, one might expect that measuring hCG in compartments within the neoplasm increases the sensitivity of marker detection. In our study, determining intact hCG and free hCGß in malignant tissue enhanced the sensitivity of this marker as compared to serum. Concentrations of intact hCG and free hCGß were significantly higher in malignant tumor tissue than in the corresponding sera samples (p<0.05;(Table 2.6),and intact hCG and free hCGß was elevated even in patients with normal serum values (23/23) using 5mIU/ml as reference value (Fig 2.5). In benign tissues, the highest concentration of intact hCG and free hCGß measured in 25 specimens was (9.5 mIU/ml), using 10mIU/ml reference value as suggested by some studies, 23/23 (100%) of the malignant samples were considered pathological and 25/25 (100%) of the benign samples were judged normal.

These data are extended to other findings that intact hCG and free hCGß in tissue might be useful for the diagnosis of the malignancies and it expression in cancer, defines the metastic aggressiveness of the tumors in which it is found. There is several documentation of the localization of hCG, hCG like material, or free hCG subunits in a variety of nontrophoblastic tissues and was extrac Table from virtually all normal and malignant human tissues[126-137]. Using immunohistochemical technique, various investigators found hCG in adenocarcinoma of large bowel[134] and uterine cervix[132], breast cancer[127],hepatoblastoma[133] ,epithelial ovarian cancers[128] ,colorectal cancer[130], Urothelial carcinoma [129],and malignant gastric tumors[131]. Yoshimoto et.al.,[163] reported that extracts of cancer tissues from stomach, liver, colon, and lung contained hCG-like material higher than normal tissue. The work of Acevedo and other authors[114-124] has shown that free hCGß express in human fetal tissue and cancer cells of different histological types and origins. Bellet et.al.,[64] demonstrated that activation occurs with the gene cluster responsible for hCGβ in breast, bladder, prostate, and thyroid cancer and suggested that methylation play a role in maintaining the active/inactive status of the gene. The stimulation of growth of several cell lines by hCG has been reported[138-141] , also resolution of the three dimensional structure of hCG had shown this hormone to be a growth factor[76][72][77] , thus cancer cells are able to regulate independently its own growth. Indeed, hCG has been shown to exert inhibitory effects on the growth of breast and prostate cell lines[199]. In the breast, some patients have increasing hCG levels, and some breast cancer tissue and human breast cell lines contain native hCG.

Several hypotheses have been proposed to explain the origin of hCG producing cells and include the following:[132]

a. Displaced gonadal cell(extragonadol choriocarcinoma).

b. Metastasis from an intrauterine or gonadal lesion

c. An evaluation from a somatic cell that underwent a morphological and functional transformation into a cell functionally similar to the trophoblast.

Table 2.2: The Values of Intact hCG and Free hCGß Levels in Sera of Malignant and Benign Gynecologic Tumors (All details are explained in the text)

Clinical categories	No. of patients	Range of intact hCG and free hCGß (mIU/ml)	Range of age (year)
Malignancy			
Intact hCG and free hCGß positive*	11	22.1-166	40-80
Intact hCG and free hCGß negative*	12	3.8-5	38-70
All patients	23	3.8-166	38-80
Benign			
Intact hCG and free hCGß positive*	7	7.3-14.4	53-67
Intact hCG and free hCGß negative*	52	3.9-5	22-65
All patients	59	3.9-14.4	22-67
Normal	30	2.5-5	20-68

*positive: patients having levels of intact hCG and hCGß above 5mIU/ml

* negative: patients having levels of intact hCG and hCGß below 5mIU/ml

Table 2.3: Preoperative Elevated Serum Levels of Intact hCG and Free hCGß in Malignant and Benign Gynecologic Tumors
(All details are Explained in the text)

Diagnosis	*Elevated/Total	%	Range (mIU/ml)	Intact hCG and Free hCGß Conc.mIU/ml (mean±S.E.M.)
Malignancy	>5mIU/ml			
Endometrial				
Adenocarcinoma	4/9	44	22.1-110.5	64.6± 41.8
*Ovarian cancer				
Serous	7/11	64	37.3-166	100.55±45.32
Mucinous	0/3	Zero		
All patients	11/23	48	22.1-166	87.6±47.9
Benign				
Adenomyosis	1/4	25	11.2	11.2
Fibromyoma	3/20	15	8.3-13.1	10.2±2.5
Endometriosis	0/3	0		
Follicular cyst	1/10	14	12.3	12.3
Serous cyst	2/9	33	10.2-14.4	12.3±3.5
Musinous cyst	0/3	0		
Dermoid cyst	0/4	0		
Poly cystic	0/6	0		
All patients	7/59	12	8.3-14.4	11.2±2.2
Normal				
Female <45 year	0/15	0		
Female >45 year	0/15	0		

*Elevated /Total: Number of patients having levels of the intact hCG and free hCGß above 5mIU/ml/total number of patients.

Table 2.4: Elevated Serum Level of Intact hCG and Free hCGß in Relation to Staging of Endometrial and Ovarian Cancers (All details are explained in the text)

Clinical Stage*	Endometrial cancer			Ovarian cancer		
	Elevated/total	%	hCG/ hCGß mean±S.E.M.	Elevated/total	%	Intact hCG and free hCGß mIU/ml mean±S.E.M
I	2/6	33.3	62.9±36.34	2/5	40	95.4±82.17
II	2/3	66.7	66.3±62.5	1/3	33.3	66.1
III				4/6	67	112.1±44.4

*FIGO classification

NS: not significant

Elevated/Total: numbers of patients having levels of intact hCG and free hCGß above 5mIU/ml/ total number of patients.

Table 2.5 : Preoperative Serum Intact hCG and Free hCGß Levels: Diagnosis of Gynecologic cancers (All details are Explained in the text)

	Uterine corpus		Ovary	
	Benign	Malignant	Benign	Malignant
No. Of patients *Positive/total	4/24	4/9	3/35	7/14
Sensitivity	100%	100%	100%	100%
Specificity	83%	44%	91%	50%
Predictive value	73%		80%	

* positive: intact hCG and free hCGß >5mIu/ml

Table 2.6: Pre and Postoperative Elevated Serum Intact hCG and Free hCGß in Gynecological Cancers (All details are explained in the text)

Time of study		No. of patient	Intact hCG and free hCGß(mIU/ml) mean±S.E.M.
Endometrial	Pre-op*	4	64.6± 41.8
	Pos-op*	2	4.7±0.14
ovarian	Pre-op	7	87.4±59.6
	Pos-op	2/4 negative	4.8±0.4
		2/4 positive	9±1.4

*pre-op. : preoperative

*pos-op. : postoperative

Table 2.7: Comparison of Levels of Intact hCG and Free hCGß in Sera and tissues of Benign and Malignant Gynecologic Cancers (All details are explained in the text)

Clinical categories	Intact hCG and free hCGß in blood		Intact hCG and free hCGß in tissue	
	No. of cases	mIu/ml mean±S.E.M.(range)	No. of cases	mIu/ml mean±S.E.M.(range)
Endometrial cancer	9	31.5±40.6 (3.8-110.5)	9	52.6±52.8(14.5-168)
Ovarian cancer	14	52.5±59.8(4.2-166)	14	79.7±74(15.2-212)
Benign tumor	25	6.3±3.2(3.9-14.4)	25	8.19±1(5.3-9.5)
Placenta	2		2	371±11(360-382)

Fig.2.2 The percentage of Elevation Intact hCG and Free hCGβ in Malignant and Benign Endometrial and Ovarian Tumors

(All details are explained in the text)

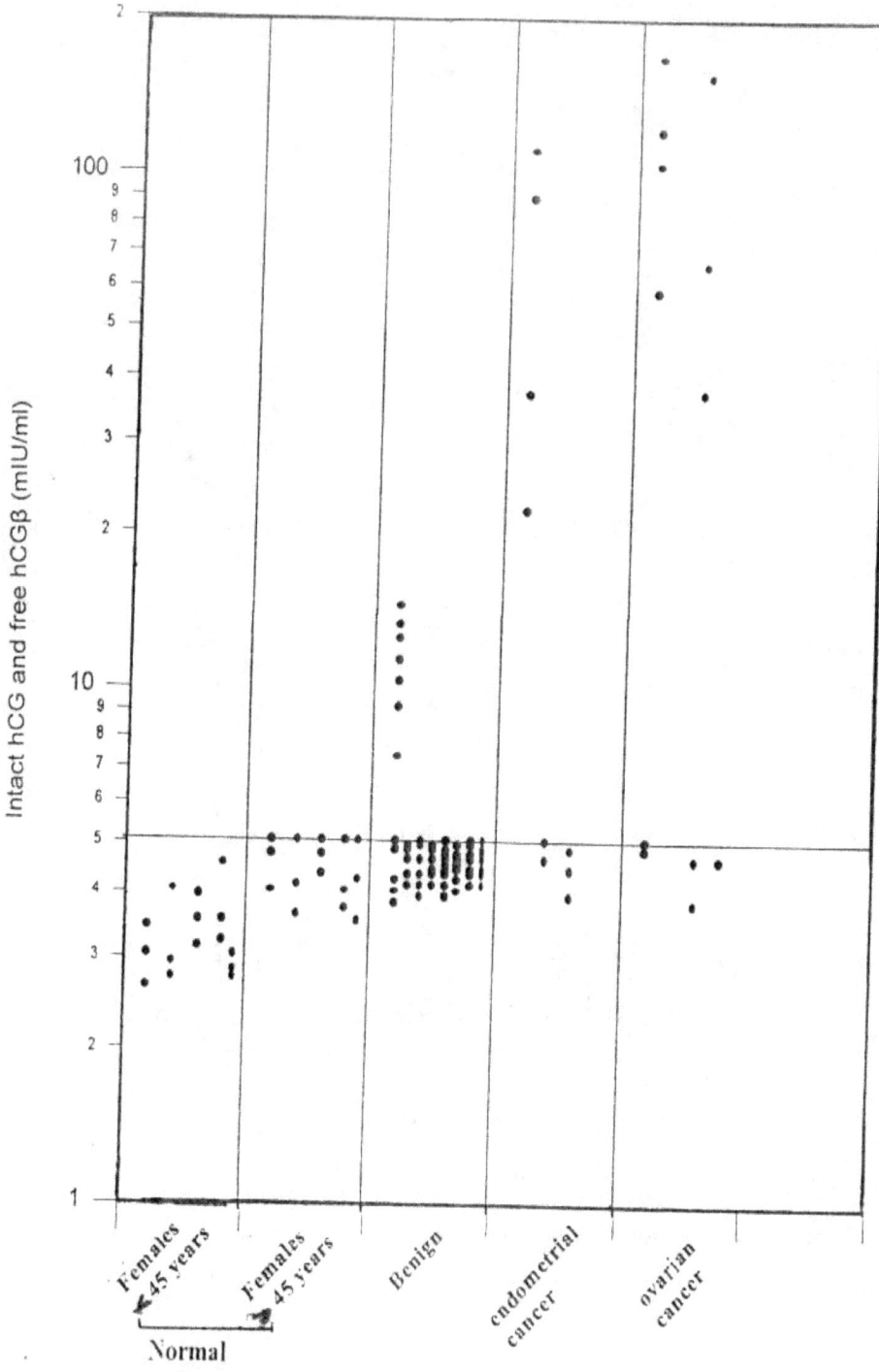

Fig. (2.3) Distribution of the intact hCG and Free hCGβ in healthy Females and in Patients with Gynecologic Tumors
(All details are explained in the text)

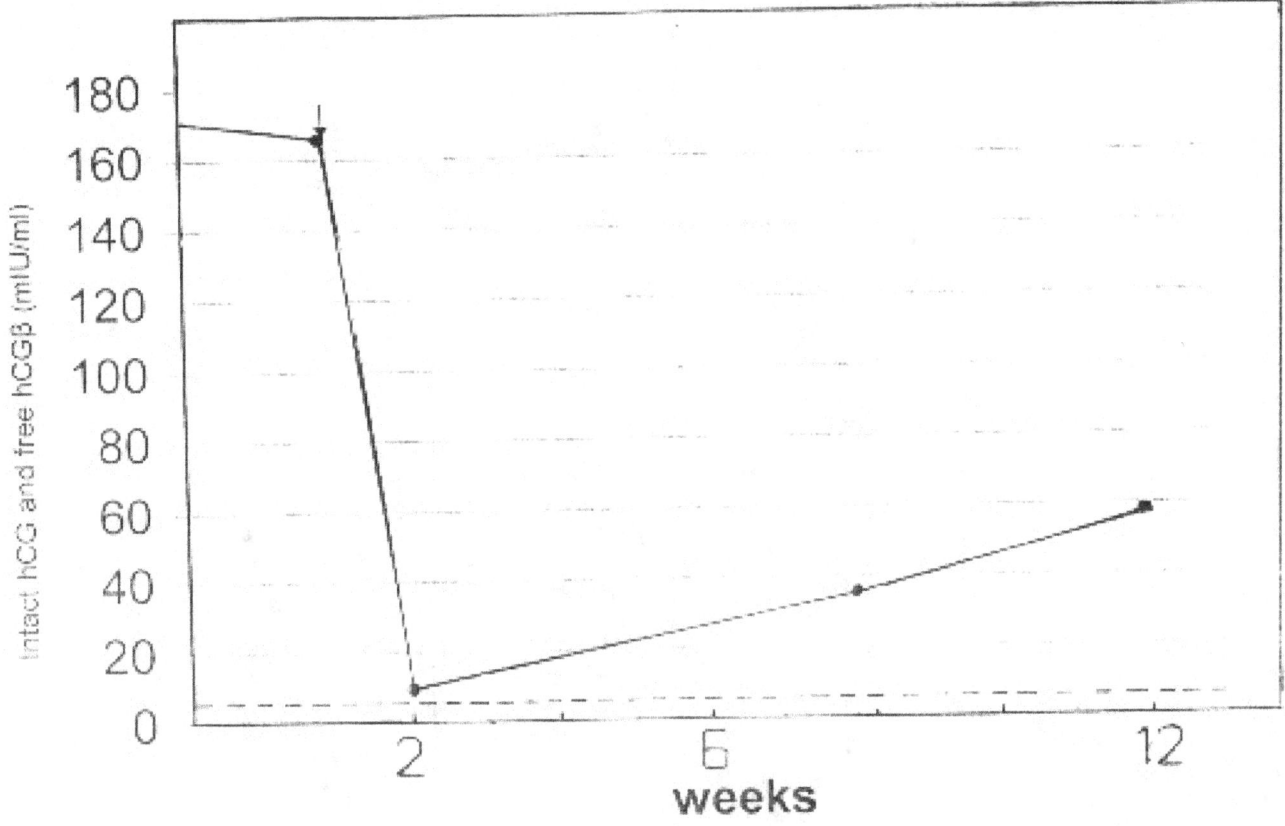

Fig (2.4) Serial Intact hCG and Free hCGβ determinations in the serum of a 45 year old women with ovarian cancer. At week 1 the tumor mass was surgically removed (arrow), with corresponding decline of the Intact hCG and free hCGβ from 166mIu/ml to 10 mIu/ml post operatively. On week 12, steadily raising Intact hCG and free hCGβ level revealed evidence of tumor, confirmed by a CT scan showing local recurrence and liver metastases

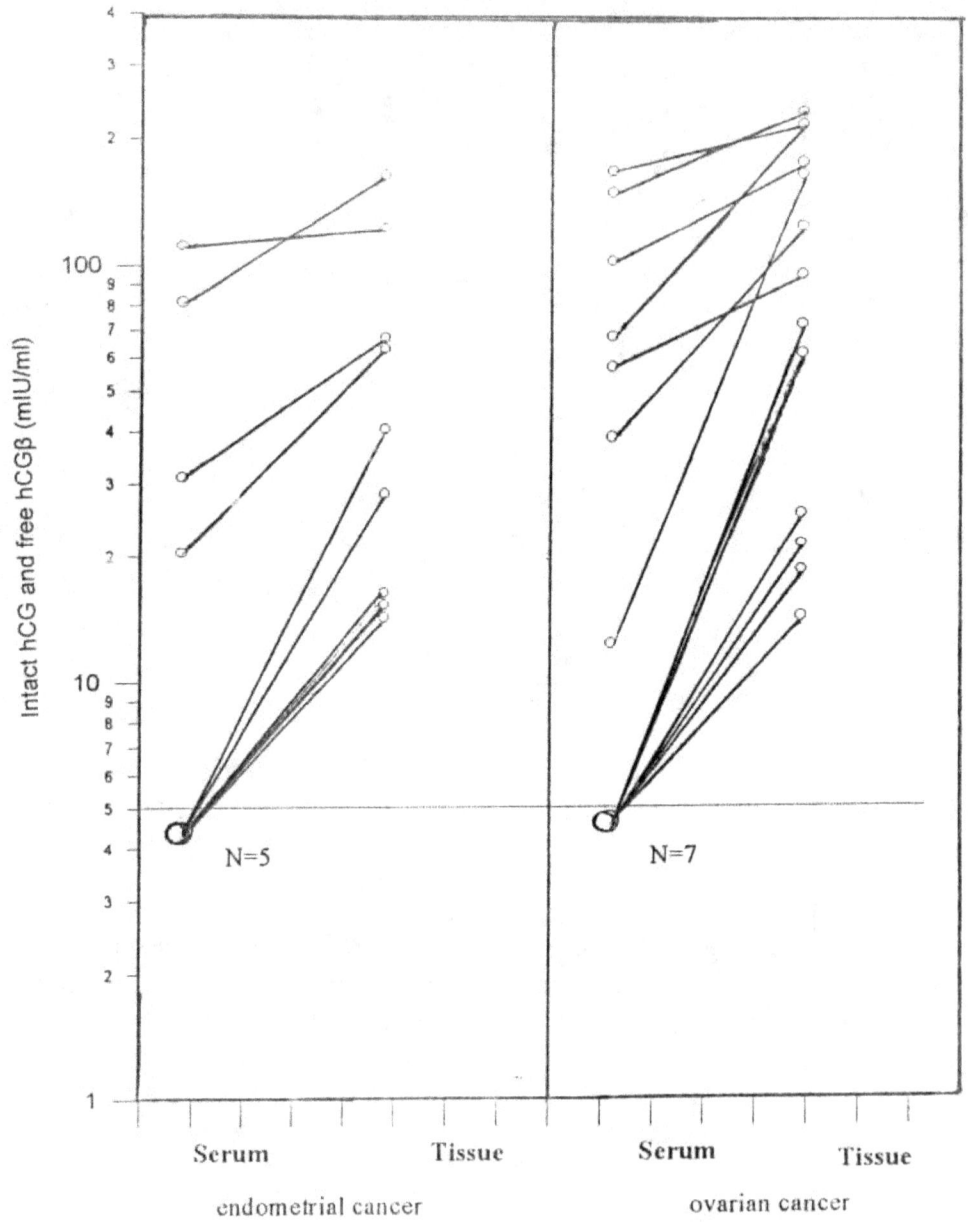

Fig. (2.5) Comparison of Intact hCG and free hCGβ Levels in tissues and corresponding sera of women with ovarian (n=14) and endometrial (n=9) cancer. The large circle give the median of values that were below normal limit (5 mIu/mL) which represented by the dashed lines
(All details are explained in the text)

Chapter Three

Development of a Radio-Receptor Assay for Detection and Analysis of hCG-Receptor in Benign and Malignant Gynecologic Tumors.

Chapter Three

Development of a Radioreceptor Assay for Detection and Analysis of hCG - Receptor in Benign and Malignant Gynecologic Tumors.

Abstract

A quantitative radioreceptor assay for detection and analysis of membrane-associated hCG-Rs of human cancer tissues of gynecologic cancers was developed by binding highly specific, and biological active radiolabeled hormone (^{125}I-hCG) to particulate membrane preparations. The optimum conditions for ^{125}I-hCG-receptor binding were obtained as follows : tracer hormone concentration (17pmol) for ovarian cancer and (4pmol) for endometrial cancer ; receptor concentration (500µg) protein for ovarian cancer and (700µg) protein for endometrial cancer;pH optimum in range between 7-7.4 for ovarian and endometrial cancers.Reaching the equilibrium for ^{125}I-hCG binding activity of the receptor is temperature dependent. The ^{125}I-hCG binding to the receptor was specifically displaced by low concentration of unlabeled hCG, malignant hCG from choriocarcinoma ,and LH.

The radiorecptor assay for 48 tissues from ovarian and uterine tumors, appeared that malignant tumors of ovarian have a specific hCG-binding activity 2 fold higher than that of benign ovarian tumors.In endometrial cancer, the binding activity for ^{125}I-hCG was lower than that in malignant and benign ovarian tumors.

Introduction:

The hCG-R belongs to the family of glycoprotein hormone G protein –coupled receptors, which also comprise TSH-R and FSH-R[149]. All three receptors are glycoprotiens containing a large extracllular leucin rich repeats (LRR), N-terminal domain with several N-linked glycosylation. A plasma membrane domain composed of seven hydrophobic α-helices ending with an intracellular C-terminus[154]. These three receptors have been shown to transduce hormone binding via coupling to the heterotrimeric Gs protein which activates adenylyl cyclase, or other G proteins that activate phosphlipase C (as assessed by measuring inositol phosphates, diacylglycerol, and / or intracellular Ca^{+2}) [151]. The mechanism of the coupling in hCG-R is different from other G protein- coupled receptors whose ligands are much smaller and intercalate among the transmembrance helices[150].

The hCG-R, which is present on gonadal cells, plays a pivotal role in reproductive physiology. Until recently, it was believed that hCG-R were only present in gonadal cells, where they regulate steroidogenesis. However, it is now known that these receptors are also expressed in human and animal uteri[178] [188] [189], human pituitary[185], skin[186] fallopian tubes[179], human placenta, fetal membranes, decidua[178], human gestational trophoblastic neoplasms, human breast[197] and breast cancer[183], endometrial and myometrial blood vessels[187] and brain[182]. These studies have shown that hCG can directly regulate the functions of nongonodal tissues indicating that the receptor are functional in these tissues.

The evidence for hCG receptors has been obtained by ligand binding measurements or immunocytochemistry using receptor –specific antibodies or evaluation the presence of hCG receptor mRNA. The traditional hCG-R binding studies involved binding a radioactive form of either the hormone itself or a biologically active analog (agonist) to membrane preparations (particulate or solubilized) of target tissues, have been used to identify and characterize the hCG-

R[154] [189] [205]. In most hCG-R binding studies, ^{125}I-labeled hCG prepared by radio iodination with chloramines or lactoperoxidase has been used. Tritium, has also been used in some studies for labeling.

The binding of LH or hCG to cell surface receptors was thought to be a reversible process, thus saturation binding experiments were performed under steady state conditions[206]. It has now become clear that the hCG-receptor interaction is much more complex and cannot be described as a simple bimolecular reaction[175]. The hormone-receptor complex is not only involved with the stimulation of adenylate cyclase, but also functions in the ligand-induced regulation of the receptors[154]. From different separation techniques of bound from free hormone, the choice was usually between centrifugation and precipitation of the hormone receptor complex[149].

The present investigation was undertaken to develop a radioreceptor assay for hCG-R determination in benign and malignant ovarian and uterine tumors. The nature of the binding was characterized by determination of the equilibrium dissociation constant (k_d), Scatchard plots, inhibition studies, and rate constants.

Materials and Methods

3.1 Buffers and Reagents:

Buffers and reagents of chapter 2 (2.4) were used in the experiments of this chapter. Other solutions used were indicated in each experiment.

3.2 Patients and Specimens:

The benign and malignant tissues of patients described in section (2.3) are included in radio receptor experiments. The crude tissue homogenates were prepared as described in section (2.4), but further centrifugation was carried out on the supernatant at 9000xg for 30min. The pellet containing the receptor, was resuspended in 50 mMTris/HcL, pH 7.4 containing 1mM PMSF and 5 mM EDTA,

20% glycerol, 0.1% BSA in ratio of 1:4 (w:v) and then homogenized and subjected for binding studies.

3.3 Binding Studies of ^{125}I-hCG with Its Receptor in Benign and Malignant Ovarian and Uterine tumors

3.3.1 Preliminary Test of hCG-R Binding:

The binding of ^{125}I-hCG to the tissue homogenates was primarily checked. The experiment was carried out in duplicate, 250µl of ovarian or uterine homogenates (700 µg protein) were incubated with 80µl of I^{125}-hCG (1 µg/ml) and the volumes were completed to 500µl with 50 mM Tris/HCL, pH 7.4 containing 0.1% BSA. Incubation was carried out at 37°C for 1hr or at 4°C for 24h. This was followed by centrifugation for 30 min at 1500xg and then decanted. The radioactivity of the bound hCG(CPM) was counted in the pellet for each tube using gamma counter. Non specific binding(NSB) was also determined by the same method in the presence of 200 fold excess of unlabelled hCG as competitor.

The specific binding (CPM) was calculated by subtraction of the radioactivity (CPM) obtained in the presence of excess of unlabelled hCG (NSB) from total binding (TB) .

SB (CPM) = TB (CPM) - NSB (CPM)

Percentage (%SB)= SB(CPM) / Total count (CPM) of the ^{125}I-hCG used in each tube X100

3.3.2 The Effect of ^{125}I-hCG Concentration on the Binding:

Increasing concentration of ^{125}I -hCG ranging from (1-20 pM) were added to 250 µL (700 µg protein) of crude ovarian or uterine homogenates with a final volume of 500 µl (completed with 50 mM Tris/ HCL, pH 7.4 containing 0.1% BSA.

After incubation for 1hr at 37°C, the bound hCG was determined as described in section (3.3.1). The specific binding (SB%) was calculated and plotted against the concentration of ^{125}I-hCG.

3.3.3 The Effect of Receptor Concentration on the Binding:

Forty microlitres of ^{125}I –hCG (lµg/mL) was added to 250 µl of increasing amount (300,400,500,600,700,800µg) of crude ovarian homogenates in a final volume of 500 µl (completed with Tris -0.1% BSA buffer pH7.4). After incubation for 1hr at 37°C, the bound hCG was determined as described in section (3.3.1) The same experiment was carried out using 250µl of increasing amount (300,400,500,600,700,800,ug protein) of uterine homogenate added to a set of tubes contained 20 µl of ^{125}I -hCG (1µg/ml) in a final volume of 500µl. The SB% was calculated and plotted against the concentration of receptor.

3.3.4 The Effect of pH on the Receptor Binding:

Two hundred fifty microliters of crude ovarian homogenates (500µg protein) were added to 40 µl (1µg/ml) of ^{125}I -hCG. The mixtures were then completed with buffers of different pH (5, 5.5, 6, 6.4, 6.8, 7, 7.2, 7.4, 7.6, 7.8, and 8.0) to 500µl. The experiment was repeated using 250 µl of crude uterine homogenates (700µg protein), added to 20 µl (1µg/mL) of ^{125}I -hCG and completed in the same manner. After incubation for 1hr at 37°C, the bound hCG was determined as mentioned in section (3.3.1).The SB% was calculated and plotted against pH .

3.3.5 Temperature Dependency of the Binding:

Fourty micro liters (1µg/ml) of ^{125}I -hCG and 250 µl (500µg protein) of crude ovarian homogenates were mixed in a final volume of 500µl (completed with Tris -0.1% BSA buffer pH 7.2) .After incubation for 1hr at different temp. (4,25,37,45°C), the bound hCG was determined as described in section (3.3.1). The experiment was repeated using 250µL of crude uterine homogenates (700 µg protein) added to 20 µL of ^{125}I -hCG and completed in the same manner. The SB% was calculated and plotted vs. the temperature of incubation.

3.3.6 Time Course of Receptor Binding

Crude ovarian homogenate (500µg protein in 250µl) was added to 40 µl (1ug/ml) of ^{125}I-hCG in a final volume of 500 µl (completed with Tris -0.1% BSA buffer PH 7.2). The tubes were incubated at 4°C. At certain time intervals (0.5, 1, 2, 6, 8, 16, 24hr), two tubes were taken and the bound hCG was estimated as mentioned in section (3.3.1). The experiment was repeated at 25, 37°C. The same protocol was repeated for the uterine homogenate using 250µl (700µg protein) of this homogenate, added to 20µl (1ug/ml) of ^{125}I-hCG. The SB% was calculated and plotted vs. the time of incubation.

3.3.7 Stability of Receptor Homogenate and Hormone Receptor Complex :

In order to investigate the effect of temperature on receptor properties, the stability of receptor homogenate and receptor – hCG complex have been measured. For measuring receptor stability, 250 µL of crude ovarian homogenates were incubated at 25°C 37°C. At certain time intervals (1, 2, 3, 4hr), two tubes from each set were taken and mixed with 40ul of ^{125}I-hCG in a final volume 0f 500µL (completed with Tris-0.1% BSA buffer PH 7.2). After incubation for 1h at 37°C, the specific activity was determined as described in section (3.3.1) . In a control (with no preincubation) ovarian homogenate , the binding assay was performed and considered 100% binding .The relative binding was plotted against preincubation time,. The same protocol was repeated for the uterine homogenate using 250 µl (700µg protein) of this homogenate.

For measuring receptor-hCG complex stability , the experiment was performed as described in section 3.3.5 at 37°C. After the evaluation of the bound hCG, the receptor-hCG complex was reincubated at three temperatures (4, 25, 37°C). Between 0 and 8hr, the remaining binding of ^{125}I-hCG was measured and the relative binding was calculated and plotted against the time of incubation.

3.3.8 Determination of the Equilibrium Binding Constants of hCG-R

Ovarian homogenate (500μg protein in 250μL were added to 40μL of increasing concentration (1-20pM) of ^{125}I-hCG with or without the addition of a 200 fold excess of unlabelled hCG in a final volume of 500 μL (completed with Tris -0.1% BSA, PH 7.2). After incubation for 1hr at 37°C, the bound hCG was determined as described in section 3.3.1. the same protocol was repeated for the uterine homogenate using 250μl (700μg protein) of this homogenate added to 20μl of increasing concentration (10-2000fM) of ^{125}I-hCG with or without the addition of a 200fold excess of unlabelled hCG. The concentration of receptors and the association constant (K_a) were determined according to Scatchard equation[205].

$B / F = B_{max} - B / K_d$ and $K_d = 1 / K_a$

Where B= the concentration of bound hCG.

    F= the concentration of free hCG.

    B_{max}= the maximum number of binding sites (binding capacity).

    K_d= equilibrium binding constant (dissociation constant).

    K_a= equilibrium binding constant (association constant).

The bound and free hCG were calculated by multiplication of the ratios specific bound (CPM) / total count (CPM) and free (CPM) / total count (CPM) with the concentration of ^{125}I-hCG respectively. The B/F was plotted vs. B. The receptor concentration and the association constant were calculated from the x-axis and the slope of the straight line respectively.

3.3.9 Specificity of Binding and Determination of IC_{50} and K_i

Ovarian homogenates (500μg in 250μl) were added to 40μl (1μg/ml) of the ^{125}I-hCG without or with the addition of increasing concentration (1-1000ng) of unlabelled hCG in a final volume of 500μl. After incubation for 1hr at 37°C, the bound hCG was determined as described in section (3.3.1). For the study of the competitive effect on the binding of uterine receptor, 250μl (700 μg protein) of this homogenate was added to 20 μl (1μg/ml) of ^{125}I-hCG without or with the increasing concentreation (5-

500ng/ml) of unlabelled hCG in a final volume of 500µl. After incubation for 1h at 37°C, the bound hCG to uterine receptor was determined and the SB% was calculated as mentioned in section 3.3.1. The experiment was repeated with different competitors [FSH, LH,TSH , Serum from choriocarcinoma] . The relative binding of ^{125}I-hCG was calculated and plotted against competitors conc., competition curves were generated and the concentration of unlabeled ligand displacing 50% of specific radioligand binding (IC_{50}) was determined. The binding affinity constant of unlabeled ligand (k_i) were also determined according to the following equation:

$$k_i = \frac{IC_{50}}{1+[L]/kd}.$$

Where [L] :the concentration of radioligand .

RESULTS AND DISCUSSION

Membrane Preparation

In a series of preliminary experiments, curde plasma membranes were prepared by centrifugation of ovarian and uterine homogenates at various centrifugal force from 3000 to 9000 xg. As expected, the recovery of the receptor increased with increased rotor speed, membranes were subsequently prepared by centrifugation at 9000xg in order to obtain maximal recovery of the receptor. The stability of the crude membrane receptor was markedly improved by supplementation of the buffer with glycerol; the hormone binding activity of the membrane extract was completely retained after storage at 4°C for at least 3 day. The proteolysis of the receptor (and/or nicking), by endogenous protease, had been inhibited by the inclusion of an inhibitor cocktail containing PMSF, and EDTA in extraction buffer.

Previous reports describing the extraction of the hCG-Rs have been based on the use of either particulate membrane or soluble membrane extract from bovine[157][158] and rat[156][207][208] gonadal tissues. Other non gonadal tissues were also used such as rat kidney and liver[208] and porcine uterus[189]. The membrane fraction was prepared by centrifugation[207][149] at various centrifugal forces. While preparation of soluble hCG-R has been base almost exclusively on the use of triton X-100[157][158][149]. Emulphogene (anonionic detergent) has also been used[156]. Ligand-receptor binding experiments can be done on membrane preparation of tissues as particulate or solubilized, in contrast purification studies have been done only on solubilized receptors.

Human Chorionic Gonadotropin Receptors in Ovarian and Uterine Tumors:

Initial studies were performed by ligand–receptor binding method; involve binding highly specific, purity, and biological active radiolabelled hCG (^{125}I-hCG) to particulate membrane preparations. The presence and binding activity of hCG-Rs in 48 cases of benign and malignant ovarian and uterine tumors were investigated (Table 3.1). The ^{125}I-hCG binding activity of the receptor after 24hr of incubation at 4°C was the same as at 37°C for 1hr, which indicates that the equilibrium of reaction was depended on the temperature. Table (3.1) shows that the malignant tumors of ovarian have a specific hCG-binding activity of 1.6±0.36 pmol/mg of protein, which is approximately 2 fold higher than that of benign tumors. In endometrial cancer, binding activity for hCG (0.2±0.15 pmol/mg of protein) is lower than that in malignant and benign ovarian tumors. Normally hCG-Rs are functional in gonad cells, where both LH and hCG regulate; through this receptor; the ovarian and testicular steroidogenesis[209] ,LH also increases ovarian blood flow in several species. Human chorionic gonadotropin and/or LH may also regulate glandular and Luminal epithelial cell functions in gonadal cells via cAMP mediation or by increasing the local synthesis of steroid hormones[210]. Crude homogenates prepared previously from ovarian of pseudo pregnant rats have a specific hCG-binding activity of 0.8-1.3 pmol/mg of protein (Bruch et.al.,[156], Shao K.[207], Segaloff et.al.,[149]) which is approximately 10 fold higher than that of homogenate prepared from porcine luteal tissue[149], rat testis[211], bovine luteal[157] [158], or mouse leydig cell tumors[149].

The high specific hCG-binding activity (1.6±0.36 pmol/mg) in ovarian tumor tissues seems to be compatible with the increasing the number of cell produced by malignant tumor. There was no obvious relation between the specific activity and staging of malignant ovarian tumor. Further studies in a greater number of patients will be necessary to determine whether the concentration of hCG-R also is correlated with aggressiveness of the tumor and the prognosis of the patients. In malignant tumor of uterus, it appeared important to detect a tumor containing hCG-Rs because most hormonal markers (including estrogen, progesterone), EGF receptors, and so-forth, are present in only a subset of the cancer[212]. Specific ^{125}I-hCG binding activity was observed for all uterine preparations (Table 3.1),revealing the presence of hCG-Rs in these tissues. Recent evidence shows that in addition to their classical endocrine effects, hCG and LH may also be ectopically synthesized and exert paracrine effects,regulating the growth of various cell types . This direct action implies the existence of the corresponding receptors in these tissues.

Reshef et.al.,[178] demonstrated for the first time the presence and cellular distribution of hCG-R in nonpregnant human uterus using specific immunostaining procedure. They obtained that the receptors are present in glandular and luminal epithelial cells and stromal cells, of endometrial, and in circular and elongated myometrial smooth muscle and in vascular smooth muscle of myometrium. Ziecik et. al.,[189] reported that all of the porcine myometria and 30% of the endometria examined contained hCG-Rs which increase from the proliferate to the secretary phase of the cycle. The physiological significant of human uterine hCG-Rs is not known, but the presence of receptors in different uterine cell types as well as differences between them suggest that hCG may regulate different functions in different cell type in the uterus. The presence of differences during the menstrual cycle suggests that these receptors are regulated by other hormones and hCG was reported to have a relaxing effect on porcine myometrium[189]. In vitro, hCG was reported to increase cAMP levels and progesterone synthesis in rat uterus[190]. Lei.et.

al.,[187] found vascular hCG-Rs mRNA transcript and receptors protein in human endometrial and myometrial, suggested that LH or hCG might directly regulate blood flow in human uterus. Evidence already exists in support of such possibilities, for example LH increases ovarian blood flow in several species[213][214]. Kornyel et.al.,[188] considered human myometrium a direct target of gonadotropin regulation because of the presence of hCG-R in this tissue. They demonstrate that hCG can directly regulate myometrial smooth muscle cells, causing hyperplasia as well as hypertrophy. Logically hCG and LH in uterine cells can make all their functions already exist in gonadal cells[215][216]. The expression of hCG-R has been reported in human endometrial carcinoma by immunocytochemistery[184]. The expression of receptor varied among individual cancers. This receptor has also been reported in breast cancer by two different monoclonal antibodies raised against human hCG-R, which allowed Meduri and his coleagues[183] to detect this receptor in cancer and benign breast lesions. They also reported that the receptor was also present in epithelial cells of normal human and sow breast.

Factors Affecting the Binding of ^{125}I-HCG with Its Receptor

A binding saturation study could be performed at a steady state when criteria of radioligand purity, minimization of nonspecific binding have been satisfied. In addition, linearity of radioligand binding to the tissue must be demonstrated and the appropriate incubation time and temperature to reach a steady state must also be determined. Thus, the investigation of these effects is quite necessary to get reliable measuring for ligand binding in the tissue.

1 The Effect of ^{125}I-hCG Concentration on the Binding

Ligand receptor binding studies usually followed the kinetics of very similar to those of classic enzyme-substrate interactions[206]. For reversible ligand receptor interactions:

$$a[L] + b[R] \frac{K+1}{K\quad 1} c[RL]$$

Where: [L]=concentration of free ligand.

[R]= concentration of unoccupied receptor sites.

[LR]= concentration of ligand-receptor complex.

K_{+1}=association rate constant.

k_{-1}=dissociation rate constant.

k_d=equilibrium binding constant $(\frac{k_{-1}}{k_{+1}})$

The classic law of mass action for enzyme-substrate interaction adapted to ligand-receptor interaction which is [LR]= $\frac{B_{max}[L]}{[L]+ Kd}$

One of the property of ligand-receptor interactions is saturability, that is, only a finite number of specific receptor sites exist per unit of tissue, usually designated B_{max}. To fulfill this criterion, various concentrations of the ^{125}I-hCG with a fixed concentration of tissue have been incubated[217]. Saturation curves for specific binding of hCG to the receptor homogenates of malignant and benign tumors are shown in Fig. 3.1.

In ovarian tumors the hCG-Rs are saturated with ^{125}I-hCG at 17 pmol and 7.8 pmol for malignant and benign conditioned respectively, while in uterine tumors, the hCG-Rs saturated with ^{125}I-hCG at 4 pmol and 2 pmol for malignant and benign conditions respectively.

2 The Effect of Receptor Concentration on the Binding:

One of methodological problems apparent involves the choice of appropriate tissue (receptor) concentration to utilize in the binding experiment[218]. The receptor concentration influences the K_d value and the linearity of radioligand binding with tissue. In order to demonstrate that, increasing concentration of homogenate were incubated with fixed concentration of ^{125}I-hCG. As shown in Fig.(3.2) the percentage of ^{125}I-hCG bound was increased linearly with increasing of receptor concentration in benign and malignant conditions. This experiment shows the homogeneity of tissue preparation from ovaries and uterus with similar affinities of labeled ligand to these tissues. Jacobs and Cuatrecases[217] pointed out that non linearity may arise if both ligand and receptor preparation are heterogeneous. This situation also arises if the nonspecific binding (to tissue, to tube, etc) is not define or too high[218]. The correct definition of nonspecific (and thus specific) binding is very important.

3 The Effect of PH on The Receptor Binding

The effect of pH on the binding is shown in Fig. 3.3. The binding of ^{125}I-hCG to the human ovary and uterus homogenates exhibited pH optimum between 7.0-7.4. It was not determined whether the decreased binding at suboptimum pH values resulted from a decrease in binding affinity, binding rate, or inactivation of the receptors. It is known that these two homogenates incubated at pH 4.5 for 1h at 37°C loses irreversibly 75% of its binding capacity. Optimum pH binding has been reported for purified hCG-R by Pandian and Bahl[158] in bovine corpus luteal plasma membrane preparation to be (7.2-7.4). Bellisario et.al.,[208] observed that the optimum pH binding of rat testis hCG-Rs was between (6.3-7.3). The binding experiments of rat ovarian receptor in previous reports have been carried out almost exclusively at pH 7.4[156][207][149].

4 Temperature Dependency of The Binding

The temperature dependency of the association of ^{125}I-hCG with it receptor isolated from malignant and benign tumors of ovary and uterus was investigated. Fig.(3.4) shows that the binding of ^{125}I-hCG to the receptor was greater at 37°C than at 4, 25 and 45°C when incubation for 1hr. when binding was carried out for 1h at 37°C, 15-30% of the ^{125}I-hCG was bounded for different tissue preparations. It seems that the hCG has high binding affinity to the receptor and need only 1hr to reach equilibrium, also seems that the equilibrium of binding depend on temperature, at 4 and 25°C need more than 1hr to give maximum binding, while at 45°C thermal inactivation of the receptor may be occur. Thus, time course experiment is important to confirm these observations. In all previous reports, binding experiments have been done either at 37°C for 1hr or at 4°C for 24hr[154].

5 Time Course of Receptor Binding

Association characteristics of ^{125}I-hCG with human homogenates were examined at different temperatures (4, 25, 37°C). As illustrated by Fig.(3.5), maximum binding with both ovarian and uterine homogenates was greater at 37°C than 25°C. Furthermore, the maximum binding that occurred after 24hr of incubation at 4°C was nearly the same as at 37°C for 1hr. When binding was carried out at 25°C, the maximum binding of ^{125}I-hCG was at (6-10hr). As shown in Fig.(3.5) incubation of ^{125}I-hCG with ovarian and uterine homogenates for time periods longer than that required for maximum binding resulted in decreased binding, the loss of binding was more rapid at 37°C than at 25°C. This inactivation process could result from inactivation of ^{125}I-hCG or the human receptor during the binding assay. The results (as shown later) from stability experiment confirmed a time-dependent loss of binding activity of receptor at various temperature. Bellisario et.al.,[208] observed partial degradation of ^{125}I-hCG occurs during the binding assay in addition to the loss of rat testis receptors activity depending on temperature and time incubation. The results from previous reports are in agreement with our results. Bruch et.al.,[156] observed that the maximum binding of ^{125}I-hCG to the rat ovarian receptor at 4°C, was after 24hr of incubation. Pandian et.al.,[158] found that the binding of ^{125}I-hCG to the bovine corpus Luteal receptor was greater at 37°C than at 4 and 25°C and the equilibrium reached in 2 to 10hr depending on the temperature. Huhtaniemi an Catt[211] observed in their work on testicular receptor that the maximum binding with ^{125}I-hCG was at 24°C for 16h.

6 Stability of Receptor Homogenate and Hormone Receptor Complex

To prove the receptor inactivation at various temperatures at time course experiment, preincubation of the ovarian and uterine homogenates at 25°C and 37°C were performed. Time-dependent loss of binding activity was shown in Fig. (3.6) for hCG-Rs at these two temperatures.

The loss of receptor activity was greater at 37°C than at 25°C and was irreversible. Preincubation of the receptor homogenates in benign and malignant conditions at 37°C and 25°C for 2hr resulted in a loss of (45-50) and (9-10) of the initial binding activity respectively. In this regard, the stability was similar to the stability observed previously with ovarian and testicular receptor[156][208].

For further investigation, the effect of temperature on receptor properties, the ^{125}I-hCG-receptor complex was reincubated at three temperature (4, 25, 37°C) and the relative binding was estimated. As shown in Fig.(3.7), hCG-receptor complex were readily dissociated at the higher temperature. Approximately, 80% of dissociation was observed at 37°C after 8hr. This result was consistent with the apparent thermal sensitivity of the crude native receptor homogenate at 37°C when incubated in the absence of hCG. The hCG binding characteristic of the receptor at 4°C was stable, while (40-45%) of performed complex were dissociated at the 25°C after 8hr Thermal sensitivity of the hCG-receptor complex has been previously observed by Bruch et.al.,[156] when they studied the dissociation of hCG receptor complex at different temperature (4, 22, 37°C). Approximately 60% of preformed complex were dissociated at 22°C while complete dissociation was observed at 37°C after 24hr.

7- Determination of the Equilibrium Binding Constants and Maximum Binding Capacity

Ligand - receptor interaction usually follow a reversible binding reactions, thus they require to be performed under steady state or equilibrium conditions. At equilibrium or steady state the rate of the forward reaction equals the rate of the reverse reaction. The equilibrium binding constant may then be defined either as an association binding constant (K_a) or as dissociation binding constant (K_d). Knowing the concentrations of ligand bound (B) and free (F) at equilibrium allow to determine of both the equilibrium binding constant (K_d) and the maximum number of binding sites (B_{max}) by Scatchard equation[206]

$$\frac{B}{F} = \frac{B_{max}}{Kd} \, B$$

the Scatchard equation allows a linear transformation of binding data so that K_d and B_{max} may readily be determined from radioligand saturation experiments, by incubating the concentrations of the radioligand with a fixed concentration of tissue receptor. A binding saturation study can then be performed over a range of radioligand concentration, from 10-20% of the estimated K_d to four to five time this value[217].

Scatchard analysis of saturation curves in our study (Fig. 3.8) indicated a single class of binding sites for hCG-R in benign and malignant tissues and, also indicated high affinity and low capacity for receptor in uterus tissue. The values of K_a of malignant and benign ovarian and uterine receptor did not alter significantly and were of the order of 10^{10} M^{-1} (Table 3.2). This result was consistent with the previous results of the determination of K_a. Bruch et.al.,[156] demonstrated that the value of K_a of the crude receptor from rat ovarian was 6.88($\pm$0.33) x 10^{10} M^{-1}. Pandian and Bahl[158] reported the value of K_a of the receptor in bovine corpus Luteal membrane, which was 4.9x10^{10} M^{-1}, while Dattatreyamurty et.al.,[157] pointed out that the value of K_a of the crude receptor did not alter from that of purified. Dufau et.al.,[219] showed the presence of a single order of binding sites with high affinity (10^{10} M^{-1}) for hCG of gonadotropin receptor of the rat testis, Bellisorio and Bahl[208] confirmed this result in their study. Keutmann[229] indicated that there was only modest increase in the association constant of the purified receptor over that was determined in crude receptor from bovine corpora lutea homogenate. ($3.28(\pm0.21) \times 10^{10}$ M^{-1}, $8.88(\pm 1.08) \times 10^{10}$ M^{-1}, respectively). Huhtaniemi and Catt[211] in their study found a differential binding affinities of rat testis hCG-R for hLH and hCG obtained that the value of K_a for hCG was 6.5×10^{10} M^{-1} where for LH was 2.25×10^{10} M^{-1}.

8 Specificity of Binding

The specificity of hCG binding was evaluated in competition experiments with unlabeled glycoprotein hormones[218]. A fixed concentration of ^{125}I-hCG was incubated with increasing concentration of unlabeled hormone, competition curves were then generated, and the concentration of unlabeled hormone displacing 50% of specific ^{125}I-hCG (IC$_{50}$), and affinity constant of unlabeled ligand (K_i) were determined.

The ^{125}I-hCG binding to the receptor was inhibited in a dose-dependent manner by the hCG (native and from serum of choriocarcinoma (chCG)) and LH (Fig.3.9). as shown in the Figure, the binding of ^{125}I-hCG by homogenates is specifically displaced by low concentration of hCG, unlabeled hCG, and LH. The curves of hCG and LH yield similar slopes.

The doses of hCG and LH that resulted in 50% displacement of the ^{125}I-hCG (IC$_{50}$) were shown in (Table 3.3). The ChCG was about (1.5-2.5) times more effective in competition for binding than native hCG. Other glycoprotein hormones such as FSH, TSH are inactive in competition for binding, with relative potency 0.014, 0.008, respectively. The binding inhibition observed with TSH and FSH may result from low level contamination with LH in these preparations. The results of competition experiments revealed a high affinity receptor sites for hCG and LH in malignant and benign homogenates, but hCG was more effective in competing with ^{125}I-hCG for binding sites than LH, this results was expected for hCG receptor, where hCG is higher affinity for these receptor as compared to LH[149]. The same binding affinities for the hCG, LH have been previously observed[156][208][158]. In addition, hCG from serum of choriocarcinoma was more effective in competing with ^{125}I-hCG than native hCG (Fig. 3.9),this may results from asialo hCG produced by malignant cells[221] . Choriocarcinoma produce tumor-specific glycosylation variant of hCG. Numerous studies have demonstrated that asilo hCG exhibited greater binding to the hCG-R than native hCG. Bellisario and Bahl[158], in their study, demonstrated that asialo hCG exhibited greater binding to the rat testis and liver homogenates than native hCG, they indicated to the presence of additional binding sites for the asialo, hormone. Bruch et.al.,[156] also obtained that asialo hCG had higher binding affinities than intact hCG to ovarian homogenate. Keutmann et.al.,[222] in their characterization of deglycosylated hCG obtained a high affinity of asialo hCG to receptor than native hCG. However, it has been believed that hCG by its carbohydrate chains bind to a lectin-like membrane component to give the biological response and remove of the terminal sialic acid enhance binding to these lectine component by decreased electrostatic repulsion[19][223].

Table 3.1 Binding activity of ^{125}I-hCG with hCG-R in particulate membrane preparations of benign and malignant ovarian and uterine tumors

(All details are explained in the text)

Crude preparation	membrane	protien mg	^{125}I-hCG Binding activity pmol(±S.E.M)	specific activity pmol/mg protein
ovary	Malignant	0.7	1.1±0.25	1.6±0.36
	Benign	0.7	0.55±0.28	0.8±0.4
uterus	Malignant	0.7	0.2±0.15	0.3±0.2
	Benign	0.7	0.08±0.014	0.11±0.2

Table 3.2 Scatchard analysis of saturation binding curves for hCG-R in ovarian and uterine homogenate.

(All details are explained in the text)

	Ovarian homogenates		Uterine homogenates	
	Benign	Malignant	Benign	Malignant
$K_d \times 10^{-10}$ (M^{-1})	0.15 (±0.06)	0.13 (±0.09)	0.13 (±0.02)	0.12 (±0.07)
$K_a \times 10^{10}$ (M^{-1})	6.6 (±1.2)	7.7 (±1.7)	7.7 (±1.0)	8.3 (±1.5)
B_{max} (pM/mg)	3.2 (±0.49)	3.6 (±0.28)	0.93 (±0.33)	1.3 (±0.3)

Table 3.3 Specificity hCG binding to the receptor.

(All details are explained in the text)

Effectors	IC$_{50}$ (ng)	Relative potency	K$_i$x10^{-12} M^{-1}
With ovarian homogenate			
hCG	2.4	1	0.78
LH	4.0	0.6	1.3
chCG	1.0	2.4	0.32
FSH	900	0.0026	290
TSH	1000	0.0024	322
With uterine homogenate			
hCG	0.95	1	0.31
LH	1.8	0.53	0.6
chCG	0.8	1.2	0.26
FSH	-	-	-
TSH	-	-	-

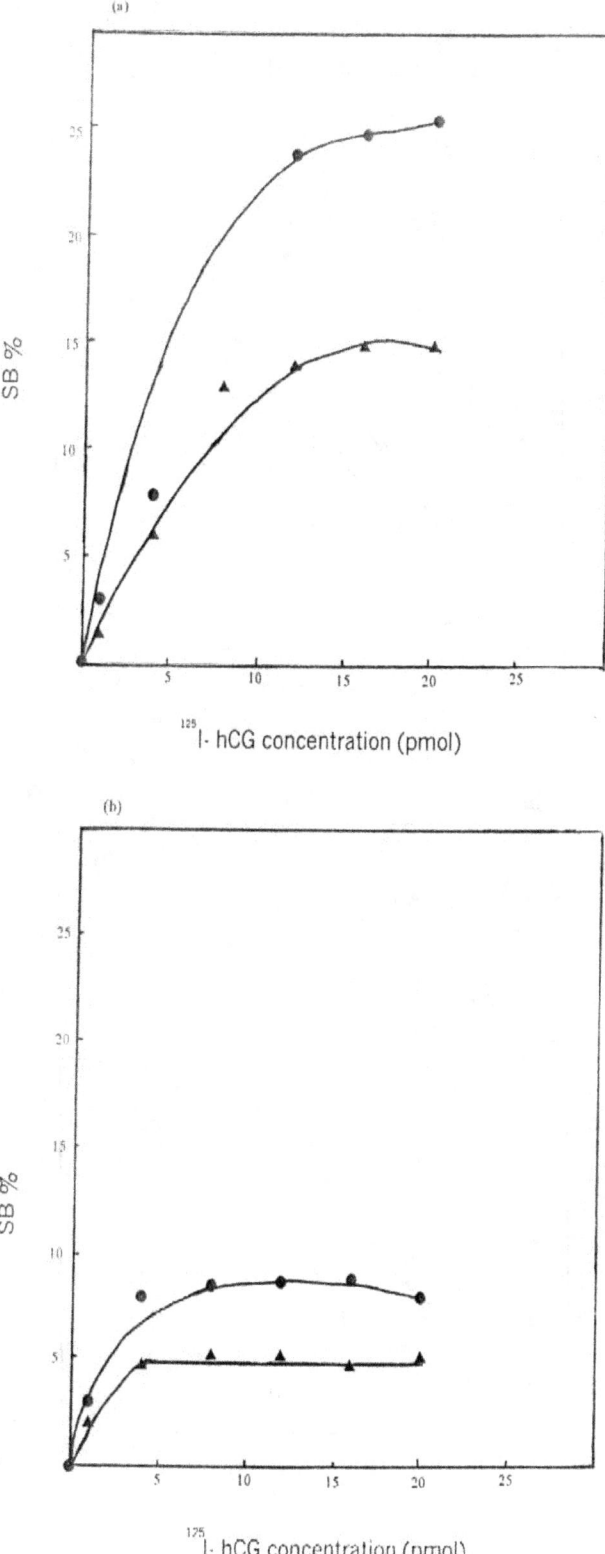

Fig 3.1 Saturation curves of ^{125}I-hCG binding to hCG receptor in curde human homogenates

(a) Ovarian homogenate :(●—●)malignant, (▲—▲)benign.
(b) Uterine homogenate :(●—●)malignant, (▲—▲)benign.

(All details are explained in the text)

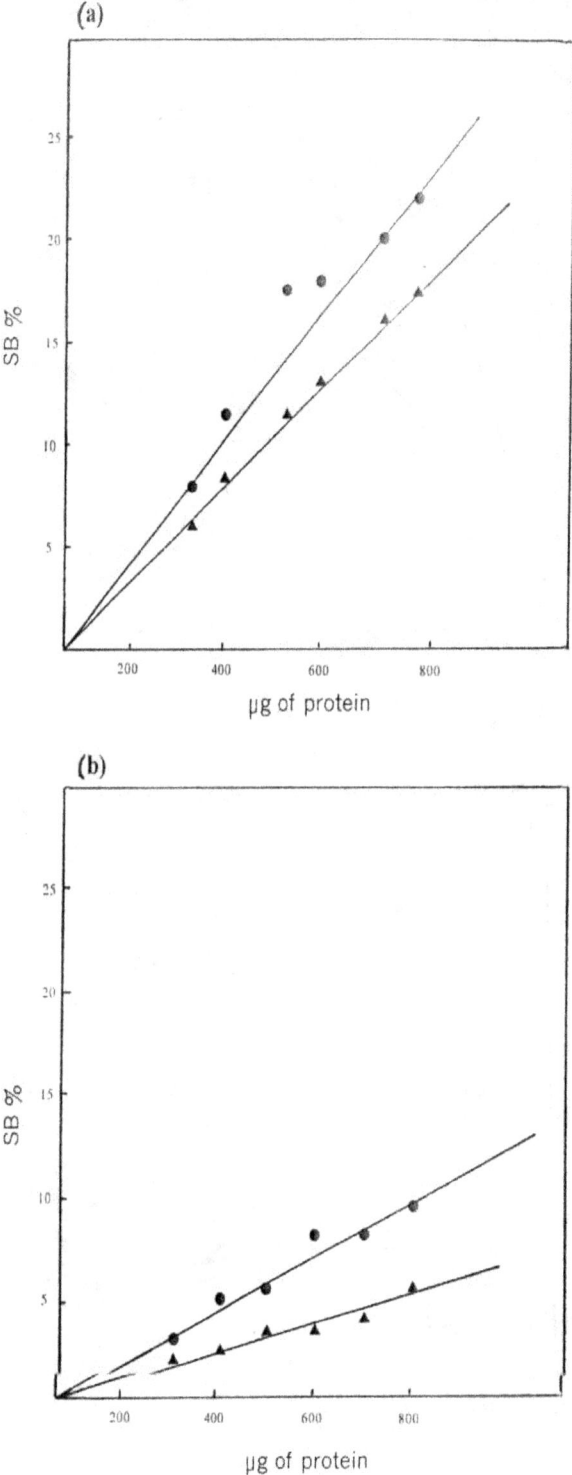

Fig 3.2 Effect of receptor concentration on the binding of ^{125}I-hCG to hCG receptor in crude homogenates.
(a) ovarian homogenate : (●—●) malignant ,(▲—▲)benign.
(b) uterin homogenate : (●—●) malignant ,(▲—▲)benign.
(All details are explained in the text)

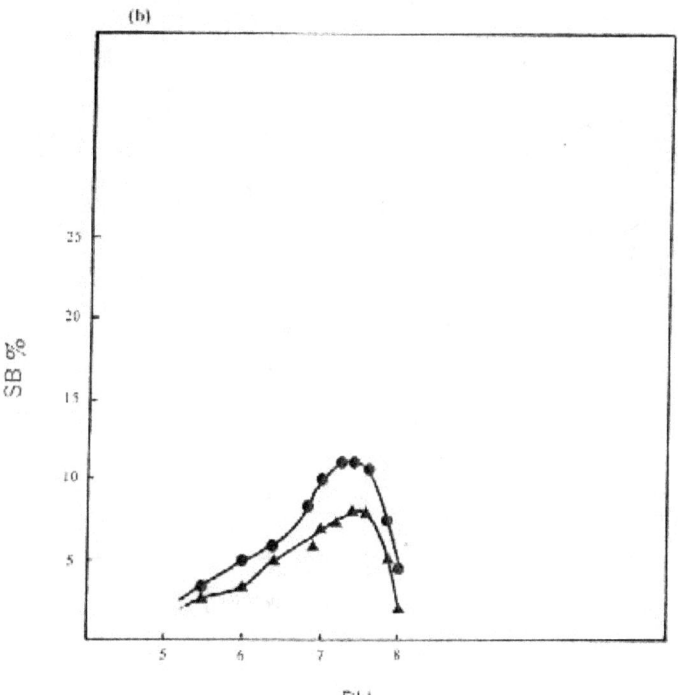

Fig 3.3 Determination of optimal PH of the binding of ^{125}I-hCG to hCG receptor in crude human homogenate
(a) ovarian homogenate : (●—●)malignant, (▲—▲)benign
(b) Uterin homogenate : (●—●)malignant, (▲—▲)benign
(All details are explained in the text)

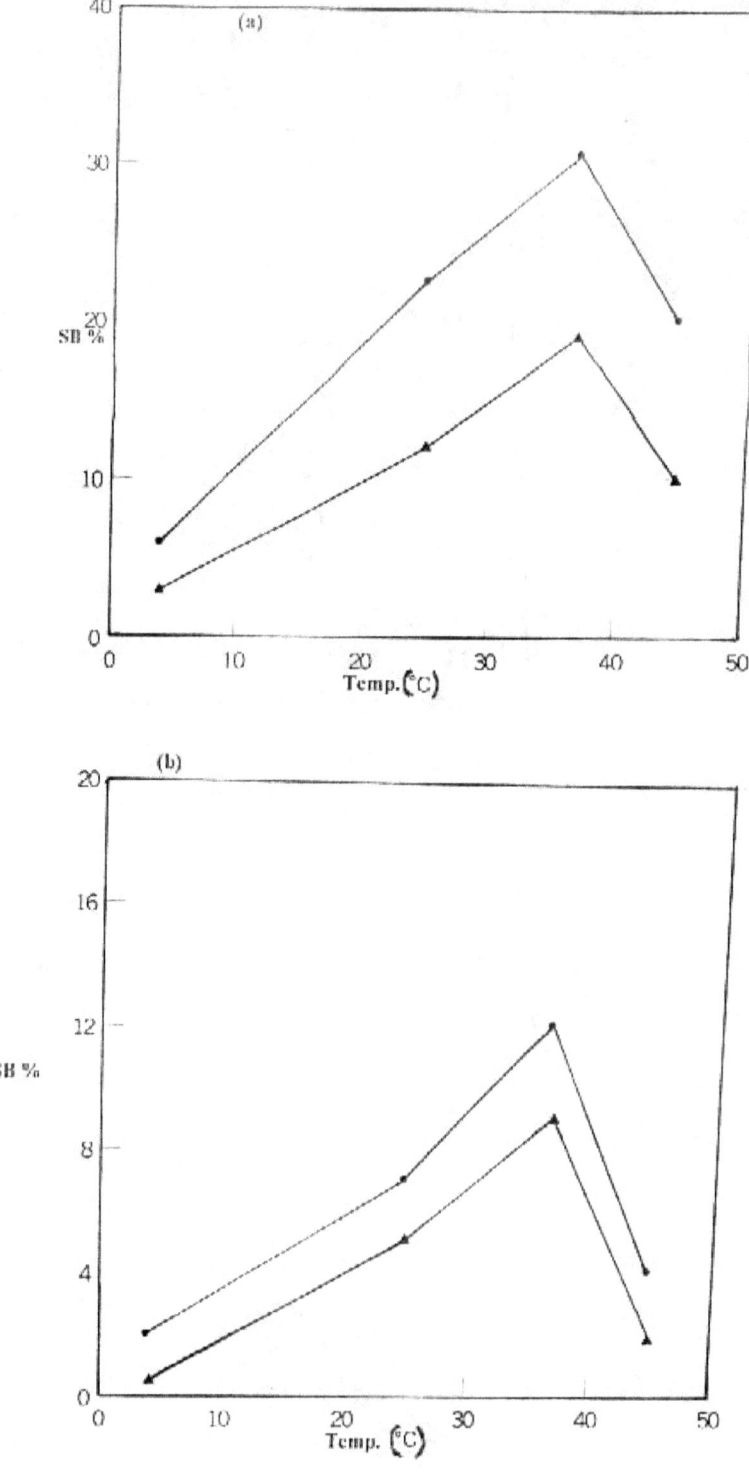

Fig. 3.4: Determination of optimal temperature of the binding of ^{125}I-hCG to hCG receptor in crude human homogenates.
(a) Ovarian homogenate : (•–•) malignant, (▲–▲) benign.
(b) Uterine homogenate : (•–•) malignant, (▲–▲) benign.
(All details are explained in the text)

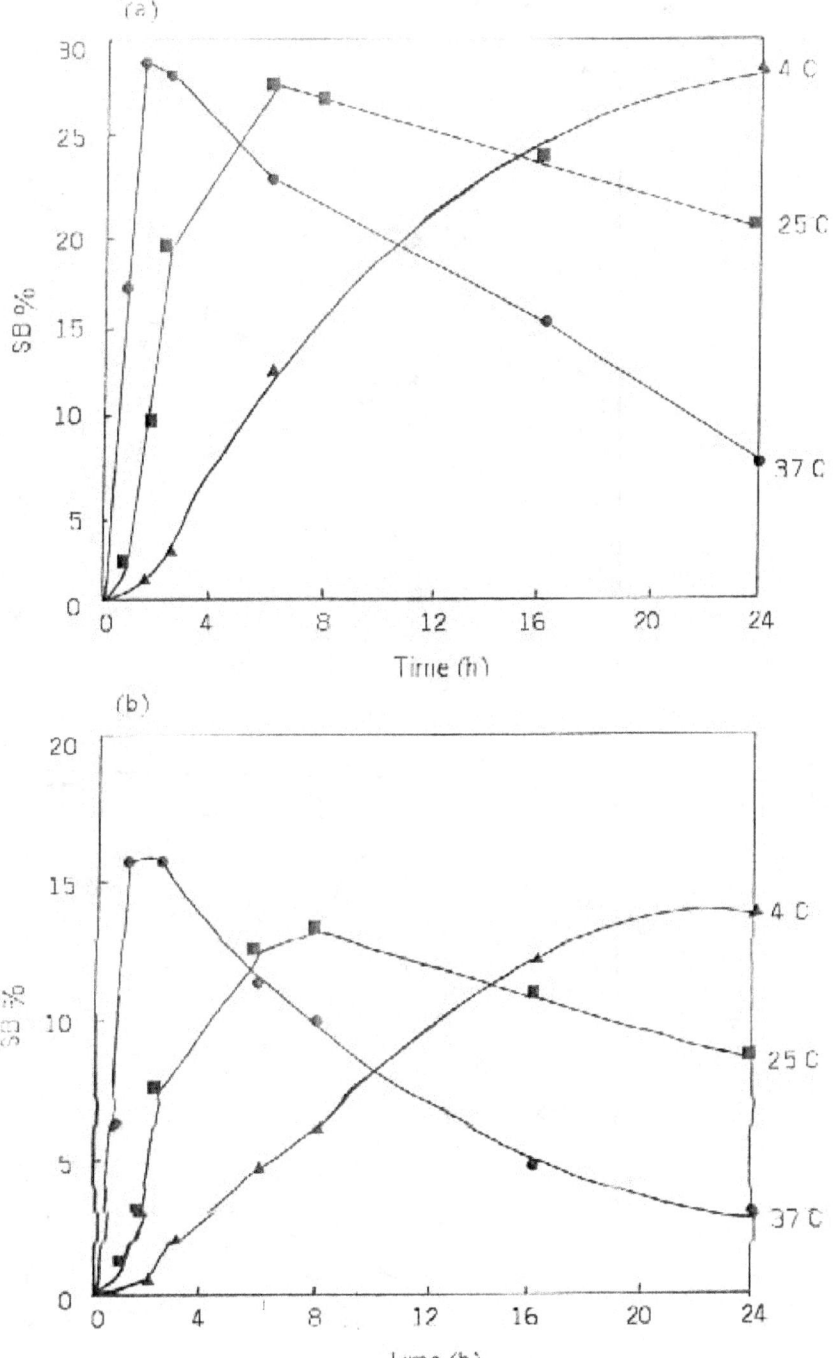

FIG. 3.5 Time course of the binding of ^{125}I-hCG to hCG receptor in crude human homogenates
    a) Ovarian homogenate: •—• mlignant at 37 °C.
                                 ■—■ mlignant at 25 °C.
                                 ▲—▲ mlignant at 4 °C.
    b) Ovarian homogenate •—• benign at 37 °C.
                                 ■—■ benign at 25 °C.
                                 ▲—▲ benign at 4 °C.

(All details are explained in the text)

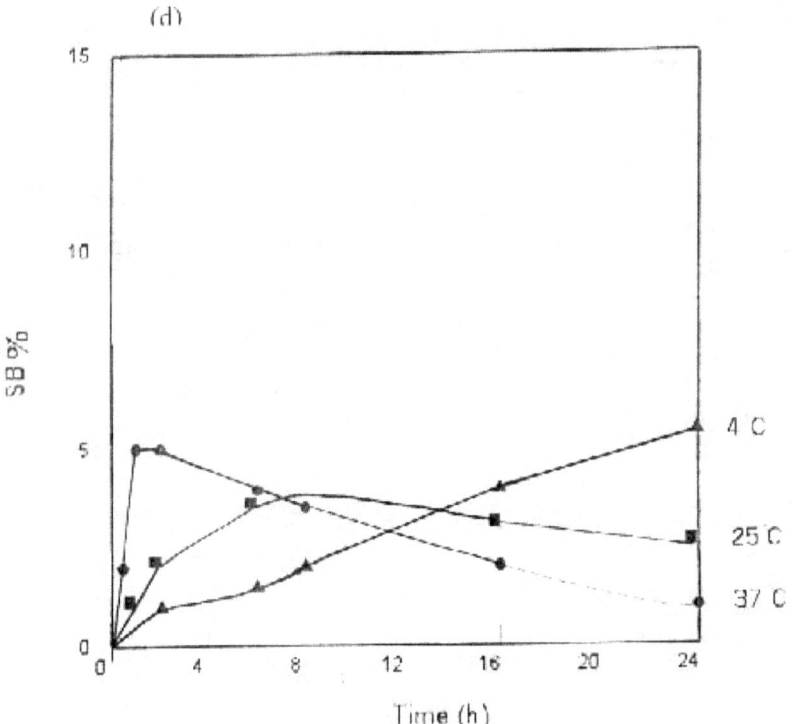

FIG. 3.5 Time course of the binding of ^{125}I-hCG to hCG receptor in crude human homogenates

c) Uterine homogenate: •—• mlignant at 37 °C.
■—■ mlignant at 25 °C.
▲—▲ mlignant at 4 °C.

d) Uterine homogenate •—• benign at 37 °C.
■—■ benign at 25 °C.
▲—▲ benign at 4 °C.

(All details are explained in the text)

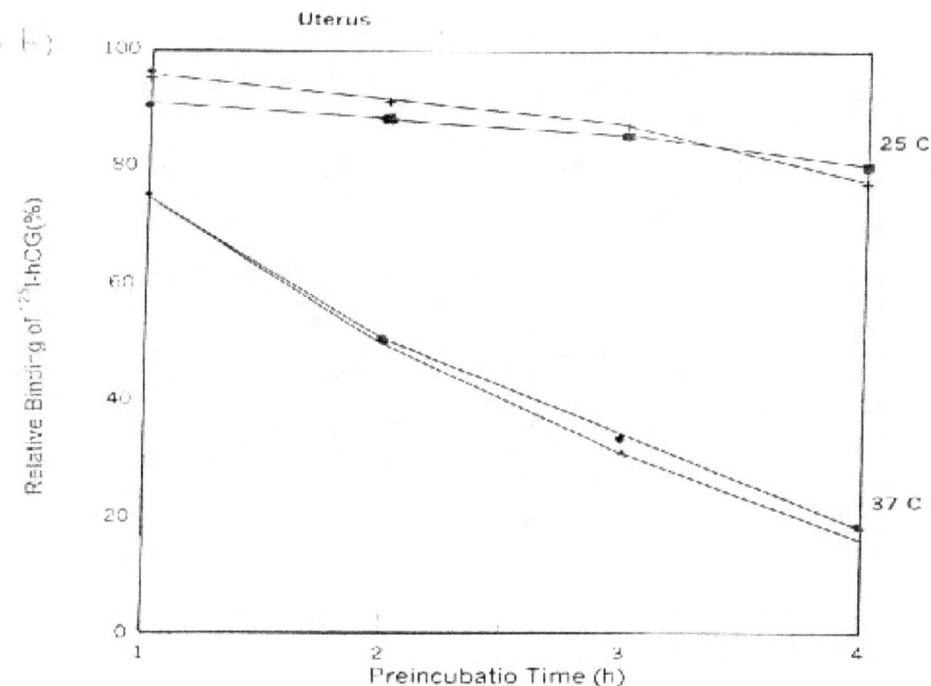

Fig. 3.6: Time dependent Loss of ^{125}I-hCG-binding to hCG receptor in human homogenates

a) ovarian homogenates
■–■ malignant at 25 °C   •–• benign at 25 °C
▲–▲ malignant at 37 °C   •–• benign at 37 °C

b) uterine homogenates
■–■ malignant at 25 °C   +–+ benign at 25 °C
▲–▲ malignant at 37 °C   •–• benign at 37 °C

(All details are explained in the text)

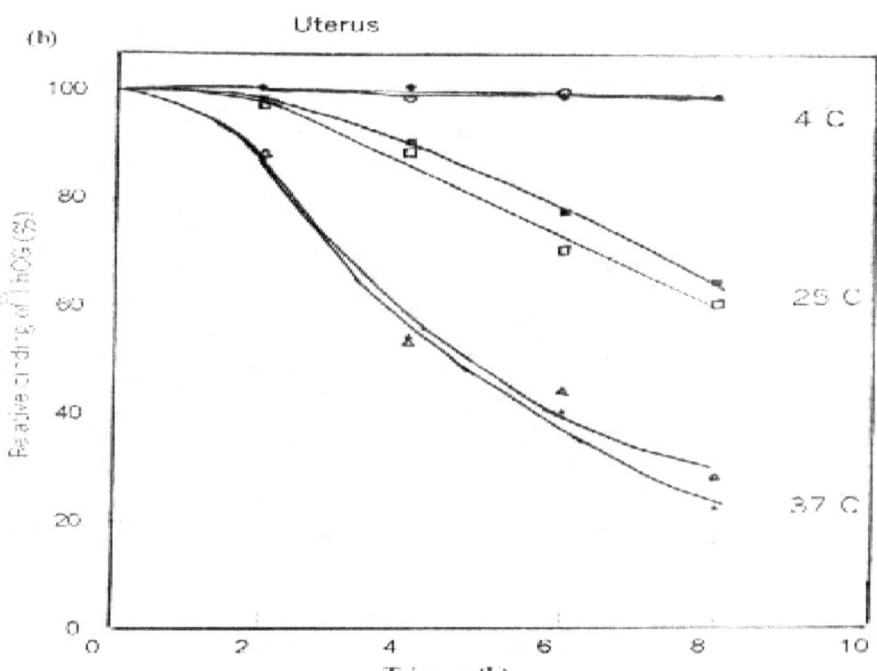

Fig. 3.7: Stability of ^{125}I-hCG receptor complex.
  a) receptor in ovarian homogenates
    •—• malignant at 4°C ○—○ benign at 4°C
    ■—■ malignant at 25 °C □—□ benign at 25 °C
    ▲—▲ malignant at 37 °C △—△ benign at 37 °C
  b) receptor in uterine homogenates
    •—• malignant at 4°C ○—○ benign at 4°C
    ■—■ malignant at 25 °C □—□ benign at 25 °C
    ▲—▲ malignant at 37 °C △—△ benign at 37 °C

Fig. 3.8. Scatchard plots analysis of ^{125}I-hCG binding to hCG receptor in crude human ovarian and uterine homogenates.
a) Ovarian homogenate: (•–•) malignant, (+–+) benign.
b) Uterine homogenate : (•–•) malignant, (+–+) benign.
(All details are explained in the text)

Fig 3.9. Competitive binding curve for ^{125}I-hCG binding to hCG receptor in crude human homogenates.
    a) Ovarian homogenate
    b) Uterine homogenate
    (All details are explained in the text)

Chapter Four

Purification and Characterization of hCG-R from Ovarian Cancer

Chapter Four

Purification and Characterization of hCG-R from Ovarian Cancer

Abstract

Human chorionic gonadotropin receptors of ovarian cancer from detergent soluble membranes extract were purified 8,538 fold. The purification scheme based on gel filtration and hCG-Sepharose affinity column. The pure receptor showed three protein components with molecular weight 80,350 D; 53,703D; 42,657D as indicated by polyacrylamide gel electophoresis under reducing conditions. Analysis of the purified receptor under nonreducing conditions showed the molecular weight 204,000D and stock's radius 54^{0}A. The pI of the purified receptor was found to be 6.4, and the carbohydrate content was found to be 8%.

Human chorionic gonadotropin binding studies demonstrated that the isolated receptor retained all the specific binding characteristics expected for the hCG-R. The stability of the receptor during solubilization was markedly improved by using 20% glycerol. Further characterization of purified receptor was obtained through the estimation of the kinetic parameters. The Hill plot data indicated that there was no cooperative between the hCG-R binding sites. The UV. studies on hCG-receptor complex indicated that conformation changes of the hCG or receptor may occurr.

Introduction

The evidences that have been accumulated show that the receptor for hCG is located on the plasma membranes of the target cells. One of the major problems in hCG-R isolation and characterization had been its presence in extremely low amounts. Nonetheless, the receptor from some animal gonads has been purified.

Receptor from leydig cells of rat testis[208][224][225], rat ovaries [225], bovine corpus luteum [157][158][226] and porcine lutea [227] tissues have been purified and characterized by binding studies with radio-iodinated gonadotropins. Some studies used the photo or radioactive labeling for receptor to facilitate its isolation and characterization [158][228]. Human chorionic gonadotropin receptor is an integral membranes glycoprotien, which requires detergent for solubilization. The detergent solubilized forms of the receptor of testis and ovary exhibit the properties of asymmetric molecules.

Different techniques have been used to purify this receptor such as sucrose density gradient ultracentrifugation[211], gel filtration, lectin affinity chromatography on wheat germ agglutinin(WGA), agarose column or on immobilized concanavalinA, hCG affinity chromatography which was performed with hCG coupled directly to cyanogen bromide-activated Sepharose[156-158][219]. The reverse immunoaffinity chromatography (using polyclonal antibodies against nonreceptor proteins by Metsikko and Rajaniemi, or by Bruch and et. al., [156]) provided a better yield of hCG-R from pseudopregnant rat ovaries, however, the final product has been biologically inactive. In general, low yield, poor stability and lack of large quantities of starting material have not permitted the isolation of the hCG-R in quantities sufficient for detailed characterization and structural studies. Metsikko and Rajaniemi (reviewed in 149), isolated a protein of Mw 100,00 by indirect immunoaffinity chromatography which was biologically inactive. In contrast, Dufau and co-workers [219] described the isolation of five species by lectin affinity chromatography ranging from Mw 12,000 to

165,000 which retained hCG binding activity. Dattatreyamurty[157] and Saxena[229] purified the hCG receptor in large quantities from bovine ovary by a complex scheme in 13% yield. They demonstrated that the bovine receptor in an oligomeric protein of Mw 280,000 composed of two disulfide linked subunits. In contrast, immunoprecipitation of the labeled receptor and chemical Crosse linking experiments with ovarian membranes[154] and isolation of cDNA for hCG receptor[149], suggest that this receptor is a single polypeptide.

In this chapter, hCG-R was purified from detergent-solubilized preparations of ovarian cancer patients by a scheme based on gel filtration and affinity chromatography on immobilized hCG. Then the purified receptor obtained has been characterized by different techniques.

Materials and Methods

4.1 Buffers and Reagents

Buffers and reagents mentioned of this chapter were mentioned in section (2.4) of this thesis. Other solutions used were indicated in each experiment.

4.2 Patients and Specimens

The ovarian cancer patients described in section (2.3) were included for hCG receptor analysis. The crude membranes pellet described in section 3.2 were pooled and used for the purification with further solubilization with 0.1% Triton X-100 (provided by BDH) in 50 mM Tris buffer pH 7.4 containing 5 mM EDTA, 1mM PMSF 20% glycerol in a volume equivalent to 1:4 for 1hr at 4°C. The resulting mixture was subjected to centrifugation at 9000 xg for 30 min The pellet was extracted again with 0.1% Triton X-100 in a volume equal to half that used in first extraction for 1hr to ensure the complete extraction of the receptor. The supernatants were combined and diluted 2-fold with the same buffer not containing detergent. The receptor activity and protein concentration were measured on this supernatant.

4.3 Protein Determination

Routine protein determination was carried out by the method of lowry et.al.,[200] The method was slightly modified for its application to solutions containing Triton X-100. Turbidity produced during the assay due to the detergent was removed by centrifugation at 3000xg and the absorbance of the clear blue-colored supernatant was read at 750 nm. The calibration curve was prepared under similar conditions using bovine serum albumin containing the same amount of Triton X-100.

4.4 Binding Assay

The soluble receptor was assayed by mixing 250ul of the receptor solution with 40µl of ^{125}I.hCG (1 µg/ml) and completed to 500µl with 50mM Tris buffer 0.1%BSA, pH 7.2. Incubation was carried out at 37°C for 1hr. This was followed by addition of 750µl of 10% polyethylene glycol in Tris buffer. After shaking well and allowing to stand at 4°C for 10min, the reaction mixture was centrifuged at 1500xg for 30 min and the radioactivity was determined in the pellet. The non specific binding was determined in the presence of 200 fold of unlabelled hCG.

4.5 Purification of hCG-R

4.5.1 Gel Filtration Chromatography on Sepharose CL-6B

Preparation of the Column

The Sepharose CL-6B (provided by pharmacia) gel was prepared by swelling it in 50 mM Tris/HCL buffer, pH 7.4, containing 1mM $MgCl_2$, 0.01% Triton X-100 (v/v). The swollen gel was packed in the column (1.5x 87cm) which was equilibrated with the same buffer.

Void Volume Determination:

The void volume (V_0) of the column was estimated by using blue dextran 2000 with concentration of 1mg/ml dissolved in Tris buffer used for equilibration. One ml of blue dextrane solution was applied to the column, and then elution was carried out with the same Tris buffer. Fractions of 2ml each were collected at a flow rate of 18ml/hr and their absorbance were measured at 600nm. The volume of the buffer that was required to elute the blue dextrane represents the void volume (44ml) of the column.

Purification Procedure

The supernatant of crude solubilized membranes (30mg of protein) was applied to the column which was eluted with the same Tris buffer used for equilibration of column. Fractions of 2ml each were collected at a flow rate of 10ml/hr. The protein localization was followed in each tube at low ultraviolet absorption of Triton x-100 (230nm), also specific binding of each fraction was calculated as described in section (4.4) and plotted against the elution volume. The fractions that contained the binding activity were pooled and protein was determined as described in section (4.3) while binding of I^{125}–hCG to the receptor with increasing amount of I^{125}–hCG (1-200pM) was determined as described in (4.4). The pooled fractions were concentrated by dialysis against polyethylene glycol for a subsequent purification steps.

4.5.2 Affinity Chromatography on Sepharose –hCG

Preparation of Sepharose –hCG

Purified hCG (1500mIU/ml) was attached directly without interposing hydrophobic extension to Sepharose 4B[158]. The hormone (0.7 mg protein) in 0.1M phosphate buffer pH 9.5 was incubated with Sepharose 4B activated with CNBr (1gm), purchased from Pharamacia for 24hr at 4°C. The amount of the unreacted protein was determined by measuring the absorbance of the supernatant at 280nm. Under these conditions, approximately 0.5 mg of protein was attached per 1gm of CNBr activated Sepharose 4B.

Fractionation of the Receptor on Sepharose –hCG

The concentrated pooled fractions obtained from gel chromatography on Sepharose Cl-6B column were applied to the Sepharose–hCG column (2x8cm) previously equilibrated with 50 mM Tris /HCL-0.01% Triton X-100, pH 7.4 at flow rate of 20ml/hr. The effluent was recycled 4 times for maximal binding. The column was washed with Tris buffer used for equilibration to remove any nonspecifically bound proteins. Subsequently the flow was stopped and the receptor was eluted by adding 8ml of 50 mM glycine buffer pH 4 containing 5 mM EDTA 1mM PMSF, 20%glycerol and suspending the column in situ. After standing 10 min, the column was drained and then eluted continuously with the glycine buffer.Fractions of 3ml were collected into tubes containing neutralization buffer (1M NH_4HCO_3, pH 8 containing 20% glycerol).The pH of the collected fractions after mixing with the neutralization buffer was 6.8-7. The individual neutralized fractions were immediately dialyzed at 4°C for 6hr against 50mM Tris/HCL pH 7.4 containing 1mM PMSF, 20% glycerol. The eluted fractions were tested for the binding activity (section 4.4), and plotted against the fraction number. The purified receptor was dialyzed against polyethylene glycol. This purification receptor preparation was used for analysis and characterization studies.

4.6 Analytical and Characterization of Purified hCG Receptor

4.6.1 Determination of the Association Constant

Fifty micro liters of purified receptor solution (0.2 µg protein) were incubated with increasing amount of I^{125} –hCG (1000-30000CpM) with or without 200 fold of hCG. The volume of incubation was completed to 500 µl by adding 50 mM of Tris buffer - 0.1% BSA, pH 7.2. The binding of I^{125} –hCG to the receptor was determined as described in (4.4). The association constant (k_a) was determined as described in section (3.3.8).

4.6.2 Analysis of Purified Receptor by Conventional PAGE

The polyacrylamide gel (7.5%) was casted by mixing 7.5 ml distilled H_2O, 33 ml solution A, 22.2 ml solution C, 3.2 ml solution D and 0.1ml TEMED. The gel slab was applied on the LKB 2117 Multiphor electrophoresis system. After pre-electrophoresis at 50mA for 30 min according to the LKB instructions[230], the samples (15µl) were loaded and concentrated for 5-10 min with a current of 20 mA. The field strength was increased to 15V/cm after the concentration step. The run continued until the band of bromophenol blue reached the gel edge. The gel was then divided into two parts. Part one was sliced to 2mm segments and the radioactivity of each segment was measured by mixing them with 100µl of 50 mM Tris buffer- 0.1% BSA pH 7.2, then sliced and cracked softly with glass rod and left for 12hr at 4°C. The mixture was centrifuged for 20 min at 1500 xg and 4°C, then the binding activity was determined as described in section (4.4). Part two of the gel slab was stained for protein by leaving the gel in the staining solution (G) for 2hr after fixing for 1h by solution (F). Distaining has been done by several changes of distaining solution (H).

Solutions:

Solution A (Tris-glycine buffer stock solution, pH 8.9): 75.1g Glycine and 2.5 g sodium azide were dissolved in 3L distilled water. The solution was titrated with Tris to pH 8.9 and made up to 5L with distilled water.

Solution B (Electrode buffer):1 part buffer stock solution plus 1 part distilled water.

Solution C (Acryl amide solution): 22.2 g Acrylamide and 0.6g Bis dissolved in 100ml of distilled water.

Solution D (Ammonium persulphate solution):150 mg Ammonium persulphate in 10 ml of distilled water.

Solution E(Bromophenol blue 0.25%): 25 mg Bromophenol blue in 10ml of Tris glycine buffer.

Solution F (Fixing solution): 57gm Tirchloroacetic acid and 17g sulphosalicylic acid were added to the mixture of 150ml methanol, and 350 ml distilled water.

Solution G (staining solution):1.25g Coomassie brilliant blue (G-250) in the solution of 227ml methanol, 227 ml distilled water and 46 ml glacial acetic acid.

Solution H (Distaining solution):1500 ml Ethanol with 500 ml acetic acid and 3000 ml of distilled water.

4.6.3 Determination of the Molecular Weight by SDS-PAGE

The polyacrylamide gel (10%) was prepared by mixing 33 ml of solution A, 29.7ml of solution C, 3.2 ml of solution D and 0.1 ml of TEMED. The samples were prepared by adding SDS to the receptor preparation in final concentration (1%) and incubated in boiling water bath for 5 min, then dialyzed against solution A. Ten micro liters of bromophenol blue and 10μL of 2-mercaptoethanol were added to 500 μl sample solution. Standard proteins were prepared according to the manufactures. The electrophoresis procedure was followed according to LKB instructions[230].

Fifteen micro liters of sample were applied to the gel slab and the run was performed using the following conditions, current 190mA, field strength 6 v/cm and total time 5h. After electrophoresis, the gel was divided into three part. Part one was sliced to 2mm Segments and treatment as mentioned in conventional PAGE (4.6.2) for binding activity .Part two of the gel slab was processed for protein staining as in section (4.6.2). Part three of the gel slab was stained for carbohydrates according to the method of segrest & Jackson [231], by leaving the gel in solution I for 2hr, then treatment with solution J for (2-3)hr, followed treatment with solution K for (2-3) hr with several changes. When the gel become colorless, it had been soaked in solution L for 1hr at dark place, followed by washing with solution K for 40 min with several change, then the gel was washed with distilled water several times until the appearing of pink bands. The relative mobility (R_m) of each standard protein and sample was measured as follows:

$$Rm = \frac{\text{Distance moved by the protien}}{\text{Distance moved by the bromophenol blue}}$$

The log M.W of the standard proteins was plotted against the R_m values and the molecular weight of hCG-R was calculated from the straight line obtained.

Solutions:

Solution A: 0.2M Tris -glycine buffer stock solution pH 7.1 containing 0.2% SDS.

Solutions (B, C, D, E, F, G, H) : As described in conventional PAGE (4.6.2).

Solution I (Fixing solution for carbohydrate) : 40ml Ethanol with 5ml glacial acetic acid and 55 ml distilled water.

Solution J (0.7% periodic acid): 1.4 gm of periodic acid in 200 ml of 5%acatic acid.

Solution K (0.2% sodium meta bisulfite): 0.4 gm of sodium meta bisulfite in 200ml of 5% acetic acid.

Solution L (Schiff reagent): 10gm of basic fuchsine was dissolved in 2L of distilled water with heating. After cooling, 200 ml of 1N HCL and 17 gm of sodium meta bisulfite were added then, followed by charcoal was added and the mixture was filtrated to take the clear solution was taken.

Standard Protein: Pharmacia electrophoresis calibration Kit for low M.W was used. The kit contains a mixture of five lyophilized purified proteins. The mixture was dissolved in 100 µL Tris -glycine buffer(A) containing 1% SDS and treated exactly as described for receptor preparation. The protein mixture consists of:

Protein	**M.W (D)**
Phosphorylase b	94,000
Albumin	67,000
Ovalbumin	43,000
Carbonic Anhydrase	30,000
Trypsin Inhibitor	20,000
Lactalbumin	14,000

4.6.4 Determination of the Molecular Weight and Stocks Radius by Gel Filtration Chromatography

The same Sepharose CL-6B column used in section 4.5.1 was calibrated for molecular weight determination. Calibration kit for high M.W (purchased from Pharmacia Fine Chemical) was used. The Kit contains six highly purified proteins individually packed.

Protein	M.W (D)
Thyroglobulin	669,000
Ferritin	440,000
Catalase	232,000
Aldolase	158,000
BSA	67,000
Ovalbumin	43,000

Standard protein were dissolved in equilibration buffer (50mM Tris /HCL pH 7.4 containing 0.1 M NaCl, and 1 mM $MgCl_2$, then applied to the column through three portions (1ml each portion). Portion 1 contained protein 1 and 3, portion 2 contained protein 2 and 5, and portion 3 contained protein 4 and 6. Elution was carried out with the same equilibration buffer at a flow rate of 22 mL/hr. The absorbance's of the fractions collected (2ml each fraction) were measured at 280nm to evaluate the elution volume. Receptor preparation was applied to column and eluted at the same conditions. The partition coefficients (K_{av}) of the standard proteins were determined using the following formula:

$$k_{av} = \frac{V_e - V_0}{V_t - V_0}$$

Where

V_0 : Void volume, V_e : Elution volume, V_t : The volume of the bed gel.

The values of Kav were plotted vs. the values of log M.wt of standard proteins. The M.wt of hCG-R was calculated from the standard curve obtained.

The stocks radius of purified receptor was calculated from the straight line obtained from plotting $(K_{av})^{1/3}$ against the stocks radius of standard protein.

Carbohydrate determination for hCG-R fractions was carried out by the method of phenol-H_2SO_4 of Dubois and et.al.,[232].

4.6.5 Determination of the Isoelectric Point (pI) of Purified Receptor.

The polyacryl amide gel (5%) containing ampholine pH range (3.5-9.5) was prepared according to Garfin[233] by mixing 31.57 distilled water, 14.8 Acrylamide solution, 12.7ml glycerol solution (25%w/v) 3.3 ml ampholyte solution (40%w/v), 3.2 ml Ammonium persulfate, 0.33ml riboflavin 5-phosphate (0.1%w/v), 0.1ml TEMED. LKB 2117 Multiphor electrophoresis system was used for this run. After soaking with electrode buffer solutions, the electrode strips were applied on their place and (20-30 µL) of samples were loaded on small filter paper equipped from LKB for this purpose. The running conditions were 1500 volts and a current of 50mA for 2hr according to the LKB instruction. After electrophoresis, the gel was divided into two parts. Part one was processed for protein staining, where the gel immersed in fixing solution for 30min then in distaining solution for 15-30 min to remove excess ampholine followed by soaking in staining solution for 1hr at room temperature .The gel was then soaked in distaining solution with several changes until a clear background was obtained. Part two was treated as mentioned in conventional PAGE (4.6.2) for binding activity.pH gradient was determined by slicing a part of the gel to 0.5cm segments. Individually each piece was soaked in 2ml distilled water and left for 24hr at 4°C, and then the pH was measured in each solution.

Solutions:

Acrylamide solution, Ammonium persulfate solution, Fixing solution ,and

Distaining solution: As described in section (4.6.2)

Anode buffer: 1M H_3PO_4

Cathode buffer: 1M NaOH

Staining solution: 0.04% Coomassie Brilliant blue G-250 in destining solution

4.6.6 Specificity of Binding for Purified Receptor

The binding of ^{125}I-hCG to purified receptor was performed as described in section (4.4) with or without the addition of increasing concentration (1-1000ng) of unlabelled hCG or LH. The effect of 1 µg quantities of (FSH, TSH, Prolactin (PRO), 5-Fluorouracil(5-Fu), Haloxan and Cisplatin) on binding activity were also performed as in section (4.4) and relative ^{125}I-hCG binding was calculated and plotted against competitors conc.

Solution

FSH,TSH,PRO:Standard hormones were provided by (DPC, USA).

5-Fu drug:250 mg/5ml ampoule provided by (Edewe, Austria,Europe).

Haloxan drug: 2g/100ml preparation provided by ASTA Medica AG,Germany

Cisplatin:50 mg/ 100ml preparation provided by ASTA Medica AG, Germany

4.6.7 U.V Spectrum of hCG, and hCG-Receptor Complex

Forty microlitres of hCG (1 µg/ml) was diluted by Tris buffer, pH 7.4 to 1ml and placed in cuvette in sample beam. The absorption spectrum was measured in the range (200-350nm). To study the hCG receptor complex, 40µL of hCG (1 µg/ml) was added to (200µL) of purified receptor and the volume was competed to 1mL with Tris buffer. The binding was performed as described in section 4.4, and the complex precipitate was redissolved in 1ml Tris buffer, pH 7.4 and placed in cuvette.The absorption spectrum was measured in the range (200-350 nm).

4.6.8 Stability of Crude and Purified Solubilized Receptor

Crude and Purified receptors were stored at -20°C for 3 month and the binding activity was measured at different time of storage as mentioned in section (4.4). The binding activity was calculated (expressed as a percentage of the binding activity of the preparation that had not been stored) and plotted against the storage periods. The effects of glycerol on the stability of the crude solubilized receptor preparation was also investigated, where the ^{125}I-hCG binding activity was determined for the storage preparation at 4°C within 24h at different concentration of glycerol (0-50%). The binding activity was calculated (% of initial) and plotted against the different glycerol concentrations.

4.6.9 Binding Kinetics of Purified Receptor

The association rate constant (k_{+1}) was estimated for purified receptor preparation by performing the experiment as explained in section (4.4) at various time intervals at 4°C up to the steady state level (B_{eq}) under pseudo first –order condition. The bound ^{125}I-hCG was plotted against the time and the data obtained was used to estimate k_{+1} by plotting $\ln[B_{eq}/(B_{eq}-B_t)]$ against versus time, where B_t: the amount of bound hormone at time t and B_{eq}: the amount of bound hormone at equilibrium. The slope of this line (K_{obs}) is related to the association (k_{+1}) rate constant, hormone concentration $[H]_T$, and receptor concentration $[R]_T$.

$$K_{obs} = K_{+1} \frac{[H]_T [R]_T}{[HR]_e}$$

The dissociation rate constant (k_{-1}) was estimated by incubating ^{125}I-hCG and purified receptor to steady state and then a 1000 fold excess of unlabeled hCG was added. Binding activity was assayed at various time in travels thereafter as in section (4.4). The $\ln B_t$ was plotted against the time where the slope of this plot is k_{-1}.

4.6.10 Estimation of Hill coefficient (n) of purified receptor

The experiment was performed as described in section (4.6.1). The equation of Hill used was

$$Log \frac{B}{(B_{max} - B)} = n \log[H] - \log K'$$

Where

n: the theoretical number of hCG binding sites per receptor molecule.

B_{max}: the maximum number of binding sites.

K': a composite constant composed of the intrinsic dissociation constant K_d and interaction factors that determine the degree to which K_d is altered.

Results and Discussion

Purification of the Receptor

In this chapter, the hCG-Rs were isolated and purification from detergent – solubilized preparation of ovarian cancer tissues. The crude homogenate (150mg of protein) obtained from (11) specimens of cancer ovarian tissues (5.2 gm) had 0.87 pmol/mg specific binding activity to ^{125}I-hCG (Table4.1). On centrifugation of crude homogenate at 9000xg, the plasma membranes were obtained at sediment, and the radio receptor assay indicated that approximately 89%(Table 4.1) of receptor was recovered in membrane pellet which was provided a significant initial step in the purification of the receptor. The ovarian hCG-R like other receptors of polypeptide hormones, such as insulin, growth hormone, prolactin, thyrotropin, follitropin, exist in particulate form as an integral part of the cell membranes which requires nonionic detergent for solubilization[226], such as Triton, deoxycholate, and Emulphogene. We used low concentration (0.1%) of Triton X-100 for solubilization. The soluble receptor obtained after two extraction was in a good yield. The insoluble material remaining after two extraction, contained (5%) of the initial activity of the membranes. Previous reports describing the extraction and solubilization of the hCG-R have been based exclusively on the use of Triton X-100 [156-158]. The high concentration of nonionic detergents were obtained to inhibit binding of ^{125}I-hCG to the receptor[157][208], which may be due to the formation of Triton x-100 micelles; but low concentration (0.1-0.25%) of the detergents, were effective in solubilizing. In an earlier study, the extracting of the lipids by treatment with ethanol , methanol, and CCl_4 had been found to destroy the activity of the receptor, which may be due to the loss of essential phosphatidylserine and phosphatidylethanolamine which may be the integral components of the hCG-R, whereas the neutral lipids may provide the matrix for the hydrophobic lipid bilayer ,where the receptors located[225][226].

The receptor could not be extracted with nonionic detergent in agood yield. The major loss of binding activity during the step of solubilization, probably due to denaturizing and not to incomplete solubilization .The inactivation of the receptor may result from conformational change during solubilization. The stability of the crude soluble receptor was markedly improved by supplementation of the extraction buffer with glycerol.

The soluble receptor was assayed by the same binding assay used for particulate receptor with difference in separation of the bound hormone from free. Usage polyethylene glycol in a a final concentration of 10% was more effective in separation ^{125}I-hCG-recptor by precipitation than centrifugation.

The solubilized hCG receptors was purified sequentially by Sepharose CL-6B gel filtration and hCG-affinity chromatography. The separate fractionation of the soluble ovarian membrane extract on Sepharose CL-6B yield identical patterns of hormone binding activity and protein separation as shown in Fig (4.1), the receptor preparation shows a single peak with hormone binding activities. The fractions with binding activity contained 27% of the initial crude receptors and the receptor was purified only about 7.4 fold (Table 4.1). Although a significant fraction of the extraneous proteins was removed only a modest increase in specific activity was obtained. Gel filtration of the solubilized hCG-R on a column of Sepharose 6B provided the major step in the separation of adenylate cyclase from the receptor molecules as confirmed by Dattatreyamurty and et.al., [157] and this indicates that the hCG binding sites (the receptor molecules) and the adenylate cyclase are physically separable entities. Dufan and et. al. [225] also found this result. The hCG binding sites are functionally independent of the adenylate cyclase and therefore represent the actual hCG-R. After the formation of the hormone receptor complex, the coupling of a adenylate cycles may occur at a specific site on the enzyme via ATP-ADP dependent G-protein[234][152]. Dattatreyamurty[157] also mentioned that, 5-nucleotidase associated with the plasma membrane proteins was effectively separated on gel filtration.

The receptor fractions from the gel filtration were further purified by affinity chromatography on Sepharose - hCG. This step yielded a single active receptor peak (Fig 4.2), indicated the homogeneity of the receptor preparation . The direct affinity chromatography was quite efficient with an 8,538-fold purification; however, the recovery of the receptor was 12%, which is consistent with other studies on the receptor. The receptor was eluted from the affinity adsorbent with 50mM glycine buffer pH 4 containing 20% glycerol, followed by immediate neutralization (Fig 4.2). Alternative method of elution was also evaluated, including 1M guanine hydrochloride [158], but this elution did not improve the recovery of the receptor from the hCG affinity column (the final recovery of purified receptor was 8%). The methods used to elute the receptor from the affinity resin are the critical point in the purification of the hCG-R. It is desirable that the elution may done quantitatively, specifically and the hCG – binding activity of the eluted receptor is preserved. Elution of the affinity column as described by different studies with brief treatment of acidic buffer at pH 4 was completely dissociated the hCG-receptor complex in ovarian membrane and did not significantly alter either the hormone binding properties of the receptor or the biological [157,225,156] activity. While elution of the bound receptor from Sepharose hCG with increasing concentration of hCG was not successful. The guanidine hydrochloride has also been used for deblocking, but the biological activity of the receptor was destroyed[158]. Thus, the elution of affinity chromatography columns with acidic buffer has been successfully employed to purify high affinity membranes receptor, such as those for insulin and prolactin in addition to hCG-R[149].

Several authors with different schemes have reported the purification of hCG-R. Bruch et.al.,[156] used reverse immunoaffinity chromatography (using immobilized antibodies to membranes proteins from receptor down–regulated ovary), and subsequent affinity purification on hCG-spharose to isolated homogeneous receptor from rat ovaries in 19% yield. Another scheme involving lectine affinity chromatography followed by hCG affinity chromatography was used by Pandian and Bahl[158] to purify the receptor from crude plasma membranes of bovine. corpus luteal .They obtained a 2.6% yield of purified hCG-R. Dufau et.al[219] purified hCG-R of the rat testis 15,000 fold after detergent extraction by a single affinity chromatography step on agarose coupled to (hCG coupled directly to CNBr –activated Sepharose, or hCG coupled to Sepharose –concanavalinA). Saxena and co-worker[229] have purified the hCG-R in large quantities from bovine ovary by a scheme involved a WGA and hCG affinity chromatography. While Dattatreyamurty et.al.,[157] isolated the hCG-R from bovine corpora homogenate by Ultracentrifugation in a stepwise sucrose density gradient, then the hCG-R fraction was solubilized in Triton X-100 and purified by gel filtration on Sephrose 6B to separate the adenylate cyclase , on sepharose 4B to separate the 5-nucleatidase activity , and on Ultragel AcA34 to remove excess Triton X-100 and to concentrated the receptor.

Analytical and Characterization of Purified Receptor

Human Chorionic Gonadotropin Binding Properties of Purified Receptor

The functional identity of the proteins isolated by affinity chromatography as hCG receptor was established by analysis of hCG binding properties. The equilibrium associated constant (Ka) was calculated from a dose-response curve using ^{125}I-hCG and a fixed amount of the purified receptor (Fig 4.3a). When data analyzed by a Scatchard plot, they indicated a single class of binding sites with an association constant of the value 9.1×10^{10} M^{-1} (Fig 4.3b). Thus, purification of the receptor was accompanied by only a modest increase in the association constant over that determined with crude receptor. This is consistent with findings of Bruch et.al., [157] pandian and Bahl[158], where the value of K_a of the receptor at various stages of purification did not alter significantly and was of the order of 10^{10} M^{-1}.

It should be pointed out that, in contrast to the crude membrane receptor, as one would expect, there is no non specific binding of ^{125}I-hCG when the purified receptor is used in the binding assay. Any radioactivity obtained in the presence of hCG is not due to nonspecific binding but is due to the nonspecific precipitation of radioactivity by polyethylene glycol.

Polyacrylamide Gel Electrophoresis

The homogeneity of the protein isolated by purification methods was evaluated by conventional gel electrophoresis using 7.5% polyacrylamide gel. Electrophoresis of fractions obtained by the purification scheme based on, gel filtration and hCG-Sepharose affinity chromatography is shown in (Fig 4.4). The electrophoresis pattern of the crude soluble membranes (lane 2) in Fig 4.4 indicates that some components of crude homogenate were separated by precipitation. Lane 3 of electrophoresis pattern (Fig4.4) represents purification of the receptor by gel filtration chromatography, this pattern is heterogeneous and indicates that this step only marginally improved the purity of receptor. The purity of the hCG receptor obtained from affinity chromatography was supported by the major protein band obtained in gel electrophoresis (Fig 4.4 Lane 4), which was migrated with Rm of 0.38. The receptor activity of protein band was confirmed by specific binding with ^{125}I-hCG. This band was observed in the crude soluble receptor preparation.

Molecular Weight of the Purified Receptor

The purified hCG receptor was analyzed by SDS-polyacrylamide gel electrophoresis and gel filtration chromatography to determine it's molecular weight.

<u>1-SDS –polyacrylamide gel electrophoresis</u>

The purified preparation (treated with 1% SDS, 2% mercaptoethanol) was separated into three protein components (Fig 4.5) with molecular weights (80,352D), (53,703D), (42,657D) obtained from a plot of Rm versus the log of the known molecular weight of protein markers (Fig 4.6). These three band suggested the presence of possible oligomers of the hCG-R, but only one protein band with Mw of (80,352D) defied as receptor by binding activity with ^{125}I-hCG. Therefore other bands may be explained by proteolysis (and or nicking) of the receptor during the experimental procedures, one must keep in mind that because the receptor binds hormone, it does not necessarily mean that it is structurally intact. Another explanation bear in mind is that the hCG receptor identified and purified could represent an hCG-binding component of the receptor and that an additional, protein(s)co purified not identified by hCG binding might be required for coupling to the Gs protein.

In view of the analysis of the purified receptor by SDS-polyacrylamide gel electrophoresis, the earlier studies indicated to the presence of multiple subunits (joined covalently or non covalently) of purified receptor of rat testis[219] (consist of a dimmer of subunits of Mwt 90,000D), bovine corpora lutea[157] (consist of 3 disulfid linked oligomers of M.wt 160,000, 57,000 and 44,000D), and rat ovaries[156] (consist of 3 subunits of M.wt 94,000, 66,000, and 55,300D). More recently, the studies of chemical cross linking of hCG to the hCG receptor (in MA-1- murine leydig tumor cells and in porcine granulose cells[149]), the studies of isolation and characterization of the cDNA for the rat luteal[235][236], porcine testicular[237] and human hCG receptors[238], the development of antibodies for this receptor[239] and the transfection studies[240] confirm that this receptor is single polypeptide. Segaloff et. al.,[149] and

Rosemblit et.al.,[236] in their purification hCG receptor from rat Luteal tissue, used binding of ^{125}I-hCG to probe blots prepared from SDS gel of the WGA - and affinity purified material from rat luteal detergent extract. They observed the presence of specific ^{125}I-hCG binding to the 93kDa protein. The blots were incubated with ^{125}I-hCG alone or together with an excess of unlabeled hCG and the runs were performed in the absence or presence of reducing agents.

The cloning and expression of the rat hCG receptor cDNA with the aid of the polymerase chain reaction using oligonucleotides based on amino acid sequences obtained from the purified rat luteal hCG–R [149] have shown that the mature receptor protein would be 674 amino acids and would be predicted to have a molecular mass of 75KD. The difference between this size and that observed for purified receptor (93KD) is presumably due to the glycoprotein nature of the receptor.

2-Gel Filtration Chromatography on Sepharose Cl-6B

The molecular weight and molecular size of the purified receptor were determined on the Sepharose CL-6B column. The elution of receptor from the column was compared with protein marker of known molecular weight. From the relationship of the logarithm of the molecular weights versus the elution volume (k_{av}) of the marker proteins (Fig 4.7), the molecular weight of the purified LH/CG-R was estimated to be (204,000)D.

The molecular size of purified receptor was also determined on a Sepharose CL-6B column. The stock's radius of the purified receptor was calculated to be (54°A) as shown in Fig 4.8

The different Mwt of purified receptor obtained by gel filtration and SDS electrophoresis may reflect a different tertiary structure of the receptor under denaturing versus non-denaturing conditions, or whether the receptor exits in the plasma membranes as a noncovalenthy associated oligmer of (80,325D). Our study and the previous studies for determination of Mw of hCG-R design on the binding of hCG to the receptor thus identified hCG-R could represent an hCG binding component of the receptor only.

In agreement with previous observation, almost all of Mw determined by gel filtration was approximately 200 KDa. Dufau et.al., and Ascoli and segaloff [241] reported the molecular weight of the nondenatured and most highly purified testicular and ovarian receptors to be in the range of 194-280 KDa. Pandian and Bahl determined the molecular size of the purified bovine luteal receptor on the Sepharose 6B column. The stock's radius of the receptor- hCG complex was 64°A. Dattatreymaurty et.al.,[157] estimated the bovine corpus Luteal receptor to be 280KDa by Sepharose 4B column. Bellisario and Bahl [208] estimated the molecular size of soluble receptor by Sepharose 6B chromatography. The distribution coefficients (Kav) of the receptor obtained from rat testis, ovaries and interstitial were 0.38 ± 0.02, 0.39, and 0.36, respectively and from bovine corpus luteum and testis were 0.41± 0.02 and 0.39 respectively.

Isoelectric Point (PI) of Purified Receptor

Isoelectric focusing technique was used for the estimation of isoelectric point (pI) of purified receptor, using polyacrylamide gel containing ampholine to give a pH gradient range from 3.5-9.6. The result shown protein band consistent with binding activity to ^{125}I-hCG (Fig 4.9), which confirm the purity of the hCG-R and that the receptor compose of a single polypeptide. The pI of the purified receptor was found to be 6.4 (Fig 4.10) by sliced the gel and measurement the pH of each segment.

Carbohydrate Composition of the Purified Receptor

The direct evidence for the association of carbohydrates with the receptor was provided by electrophoresis analysis, where the band identified as receptor gave positive stained for Schiff reagent, and by carbohydrate determination was 8%.

All groups of investigators reported a fact that the hCG-R is a glycoprotein[158]. Indirect evidence for the association of carbohydrates with receptor have been provided by binding of the receptor to concanavalin A during affinity purifications[158][219]. Dattateryamurty et.al.,[157] shown the total carbohydrate content of the receptor fraction was 10%, mannose and galactose were the predominant hexoses and the carbohydrate moiety of the receptor contained both N-acetylglucosamine as well as sialic acid. The six potential sites for N-linked glycosylation on extracellular domine of the receptor were proposed from experiments of cloning of cDNA using oligonucleocides based on amino acid sequences obtained from the purified rat Luteal hCG-R[2]. The possible involvement of the carbohydrate moieties of the receptor in the recognition and high affinity binding of hCG have been examined using different approaches. All groups of investigators reported that neuraminidase treatment reduced the molecular mass of the hCG-R without affecting its ability to bind hormone[242][243]. In more recent studies, introduced mutation in each of the six N-linked glycosylation and tested for the effects of these mutations on hCG binding [244][245].

The conclusion of these studies, shows that at least one of the carbohydrate chains of the hCG receptor is needed for hCG binding and carbohydrate may be important for proper trafficking of receptor to the plasma membranes.

Human Chorionic Gonadotropin Binding Specificity of Purified Receptor

The specificity of hCG binding of purified receptor was evaluated in competition experiments with unlabeled glycoprotein hormones, prolactin, and drugs used in chemotherapy (5-Fu, haloxa, and cisplatin. The ^{125}I-hCG binding of the purified receptor was inhibited in a dose-dependent manner by the unlabeled hCG and LH(Fig 4.11). The purified soluble receptor has specificity similar to those of the crude membranes receptor and the expected rank order of binding affinities for the LH and hCG was retained in the purified material.

At the level up to 1mg, no inhibition was observed with FSH, TSH, Prolactin and cytotoxic antineoplastic agents. These results indicate that the purified receptor retains it hormonal specificity and has no significant cross-reaction with other peptide

, glycoprotein, and the cytotoxic agents which used for first treatment of cancer or for second line treatment as single or combination to kill cancer cell in the body after surgery to control tumor growth[13][16] .Also showed no effect on hCG binding activity of the purified receptor.

The UV-Spectrum of hCG and hCG-Receptor Complex

The UV spectrum of hCG and hCG-receptor complex were measured to determine their maximum wavelengths, and the alteration in the UV spectra as a result of their interaction.

As shown in Fig 4.12, the spectrum of hCG consisted of two maximum wavelength, λ_{max1} at 275.0 nm with an absorbance 2.159 and λ_{max2} at 231.2 nm with an absorbance 2.359. The ultraviolet absorption spectrum of protein solution in the region (250-310) nm are contributed mainly from phenylalanyle, trosyl, and tryptophanyl residues. At shorter wave lengths contribution comes from other group such as histidyl residues and the peptide [246][247] bonds. Changes in the environment of these chromophores (e.g. pH, temp, ionic strength, solvent etc...) can lead to alteration in the absorption spectrum, also configurational changes of the protein may be also involved environmental changes. The UV spectrum of hCG-receptor complex is illustrated in Fig (4.13), The spectrum consisted of one maximum wavelength at 219nm with an absorbance 1.81 and the λ_{max1} 275 for the hCG was disappeared . Protein shows a strong absorption in the range 180-220nm, which arises from electronic transition in the polypeptide backbone itself and is therefore sensitive to backbone conformation. When the hCG and receptor associated, chromphores may be buried at the newly formed interface or conformational changes of the hormone or receptor may bury previously exposed chromophores [246] .These proposals agree with studies on hCG receptor interaction which indicate, to the prescience of multiple contact sites between the exodomain of the receptor and both subunits of hCG [164][166], and conformational changes for both hCG and receptor[158][175-177].

Stability of Purified Receptor

The crude and purified receptor were stored at -20°C in glycerol-containing media for about 3 month to study the stability of this receptor and to check it efficiencies of binding throughout the storage period every one weak. The results in Fig 4.14 demonstrate that the crude receptor was more stable than purified receptor. The purified receptor was stable for about 2 months while the binding activity of the crude receptor was remained without significant changes for more than two months.

To obtain the stabilization of the crude solubilized receptor by glycerol, receptor (extracted with 0.1% Triton X-100) containing (0-50%) glycerol were tested. The data in Fig 4.15 show that the binding activity of the solubilized receptor is maximal when concentration of glycerol of 20% or greater are utilized. As shown in Fig 4.15 there is 70% loss in binding activity of the receptor during storage at 4°C within 24h in the absence of glycerol. The instability of the soluble receptor was not dependent on prior storage of the tissue or the concentration of Triton X-100. In contrast if glycerol (20% or greater) is included in the same incubation, there is only a 5-10% loss in binding activity. Therefore the receptor must be maintained in glycerol (of at least 20%) to preserve its binding activity actually 20% glycerol was included in all buffer used to solubilize and store hCG-recptor preparation. Previous studies also used glycerol to obtain stable preparation of the crude soluble receptor from bovine corpus luteal[157], rat testis and rat ovary[156][208]. Glycerol may stabilized the receptor by favoring a thermodynamically stable conformation in solution by sequestration of hydrophobic amino acids from the solvent[248]. Furthermore. It had been shown that the hCG receptor complex is considerably more stable than the native receptor even in crude preparation[248].

In addition, Bruch et.al.,[156] have found that the regulatory and catalytic component of adenylate cyclase system also appears to be stable in the presence of glycerol

Kinetic of Purified Receptor Binding and the Determination of Hill Coefficient

The kinetics of ^{125}I-hCG binding to the purified receptor were examined at 4°C under the condition of radioreceptor assay. Accurate binding parameters could not be obtained at higher temperatures, apparently as a consequence of thermal inactivation of the receptor. However, at 4°C, bound hCG was assayed at various time intervals up to the steady state level. The binding of ^{125}I-hCG to the receptor reached a stable maximum after 24hr of incubation (Fig 4.16a). Addition of excess unlabeled hCG to preformed ^{125}I-hCG receptor complexes partially reversed the binding of the labeled hCG resulting in the dissociation of approximately 80% of the preformed hCG receptor complexes (Fig 4.16 a) .The time course data for the association and dissociation process were analyzed by the pseudo first orders and first order kinetic models, used previously to characterize the hCG binding kinetics of purified hCG receptor preparation [156].

The rate of formation of hCG receptor complex was linear over the first 8h of the time course (Fig 4.16b). In contrast, the kinetics of dissociation were biphasic and were characterized by an initial rapid phase followed by a much slower rate of dissociation (Fig 4.16c). The biphasic nature of the dissociation kinetics has been previously observed with crude and purified preparation of the hCG receptor[156][218]. The rate constants for association and dissociation determined with the purified receptor and the equilibrium binding constant calculated from the kinetic parameters are shown in Table (4.2). The equilibrium binding constants calculated from the kinetic parameters were in good agreement with those determined by Scatchard analysis.

The dissociation rate constant (k_{-1}) was estimated by incubating ^{125}I-hCG and receptor for a given period of time and then infinite dilution for ^{125}I-hCG concentration was performed by adding excess of unlabeled hCG. Negative cooperatively may be a part of the binding process when unlabeled hormone accelerates the dissociation rate, but when the receptor site concentration approaches or exceeds K_d of the ^{125}I-hCG, diffusion of dissociated ^{125}I-hCG away from free receptor sites is progressively hampered probably because of the very high local concentrations of unoccupied binding sites.

The Hill plot analysis was carried out in order to determine the Hill coefficient. The result revealed that this coefficient was equal to 1 (Fig 4.17) suggesting that there was no cooperatively during the binding reaction.

Table 4.1 Purification of the hCG receptor from ovarian cancer(All details are explained in the text)

Step	Protein (mg)	^{125}I-hCG binding(pmol)	Specific activity (pmol/mg)	Purification fold	Recovery %
Homogenate	150	130.2	0.87	1	100
Crude membrane	90	115.6	1.28	1.72	89
Soluble extract	30	51.2	1.71	1.95	39
Sepharose Cl6B	5.6	35.7	6.38	7.36	27
hCG-Sepharose	2.1 (µg)	15.6	7.43	8,538	12

Table 4.2 Kinetic and equilibrium hCG binding constants for the purified receptor.

*k_a (×10^7 m^{-1}.min^{-1})	7.6
*k_d (×10^{-3} (min^{-1}))	2.78
*K_a (×10^9 m^{-1})	
Kinetics	27.33
equilibrium	91.0

k_a: pseudo first –order constant for hCG receptor complex formation

k_d: first –order constant for hCG –receptor complex dissociation

Ka: equilibrium association constant estimated from k_a/k_d (kinetics) or Scatchard analysis (equilibrium)

Fig 4.1 Fractionation of soluble receptor on Sepharose CL6B

(0---0) Absorbance at 230 nm
(   ) SB%
(All details are explained in the text)

Fig 4.2 Elution of the rceptor from hCG-Sepharose affinity column

(All details are explained in the text)

Fig.4.4 conventional- PAGE (7.5%) of Crude and purified hCG receptor in different steps of purification.

Lane 1 Crude hCG receptors homogenate

Lane 2 Crude membranes homogenate

Lane 3 Fractions obtained by gel filtration chromatography

Lane 4 Fractions obtained by affinity chromatography

(All details are explained in the text)

Fig 4.5 SDS –PAGE of purified hCG receptor.

(All details are explained in the text)

Fig   Calbration Curve for determination of M.wt of the purified hCG receptor by SDS-PAGE(10%)

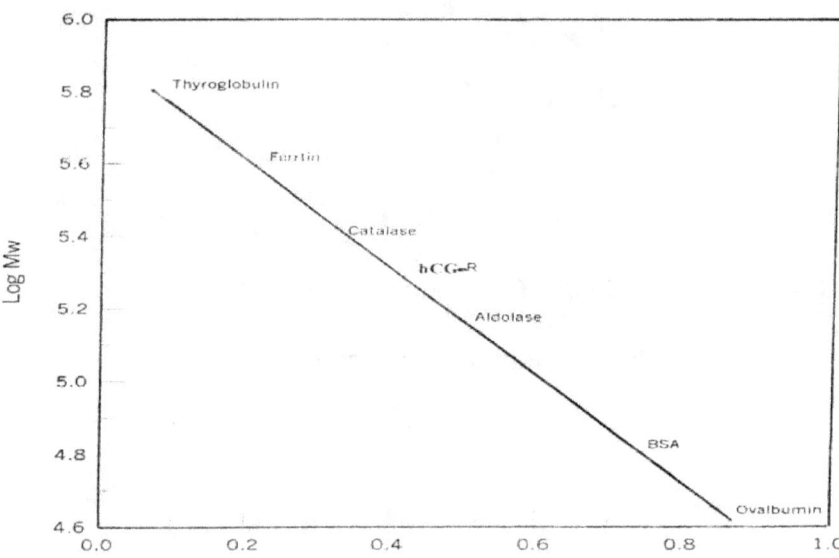

Fig   Calibration Curve for determination of M.wt of the purified hCG receptor By gel filtration chromatography.

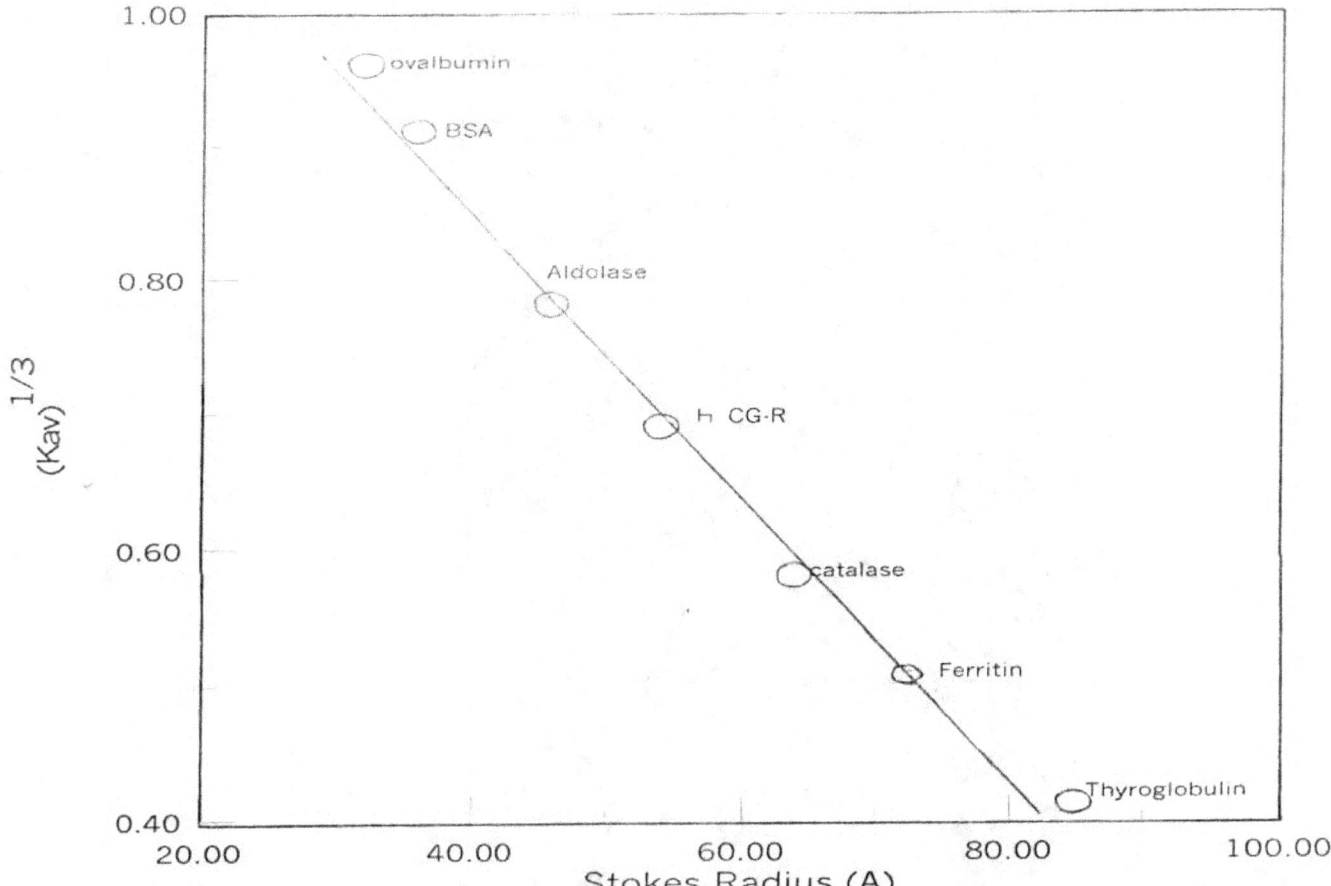

Fig Calibration curve for determination of molecular siz of the purified receptor by gel filtration chomatography

Fig 4.9 Isoelectric focusing of purified hCG receptor
(All details are explained in the text)

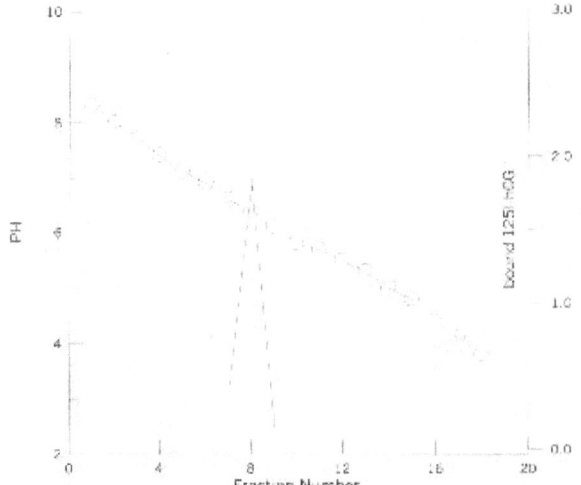

Fig 4.10 PH gradient in isoelectric focusing of purified receptor
(All details are explained in the text)

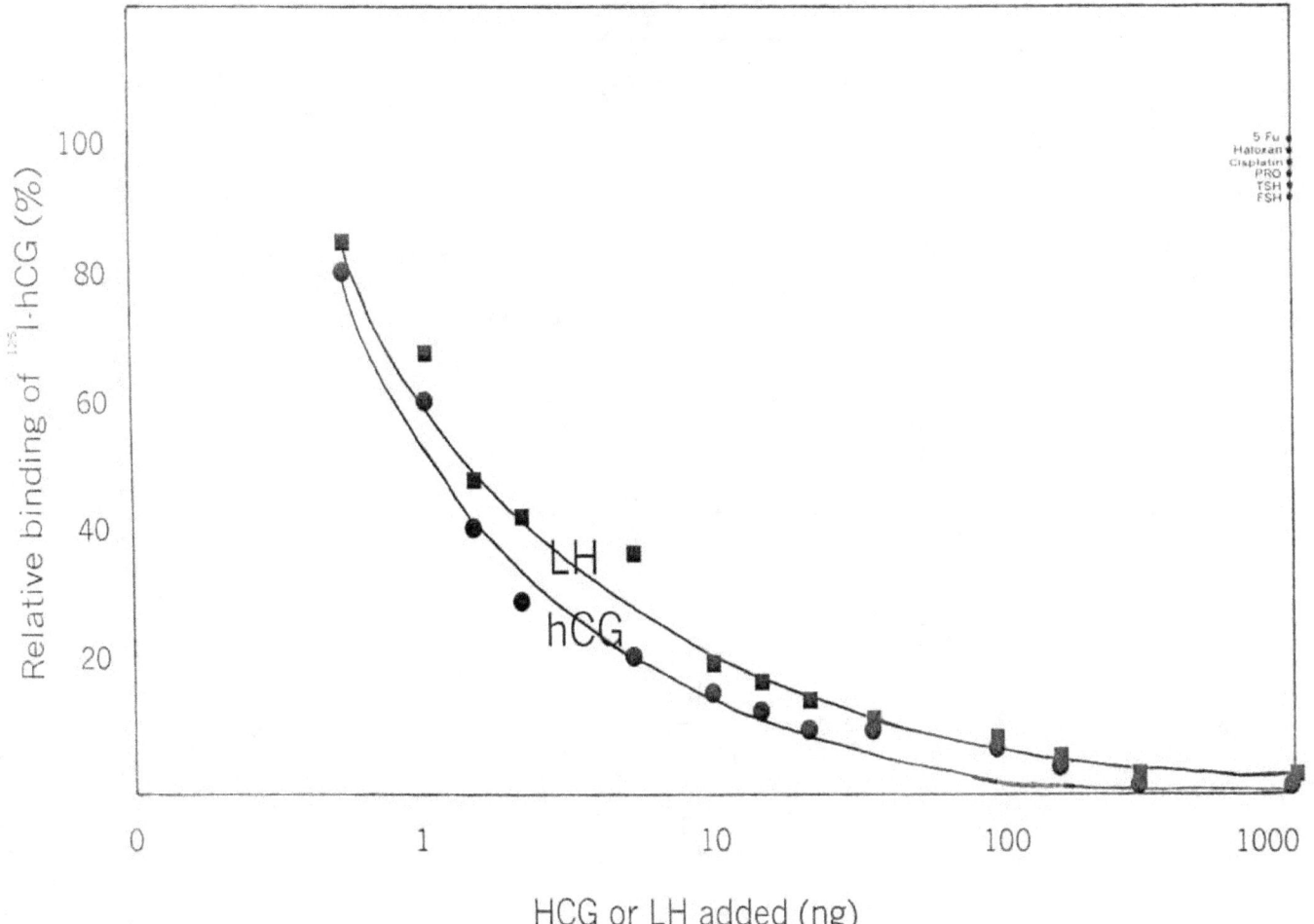

Fig inhibition of ^{125}I·hCG binding with purified hCG receptor by addition of increasing concentration of unlabeled hCG and LH. The effect of 1μg of FSH, TSH, PRO, 5-FU, Haloxan, and Cispltin are also shown

Fig   The UV Spectrum of hCG

Fig   The UV Spectrum of hCG-Receptor complex

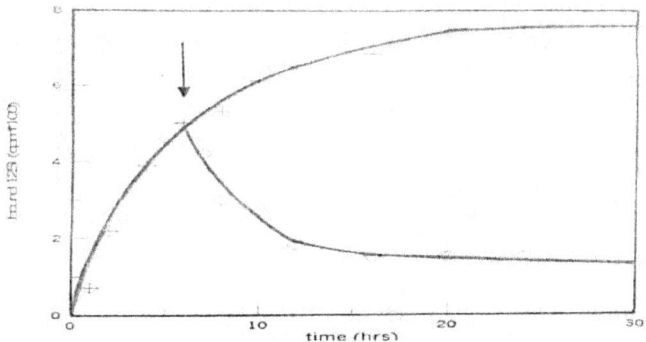

a- Time course of ^{125}I- hCG binding to the purified receptor. At the point indicated by the arrow, excess unlabeled hCG (1 µg) was added to obtain the dissociation time course

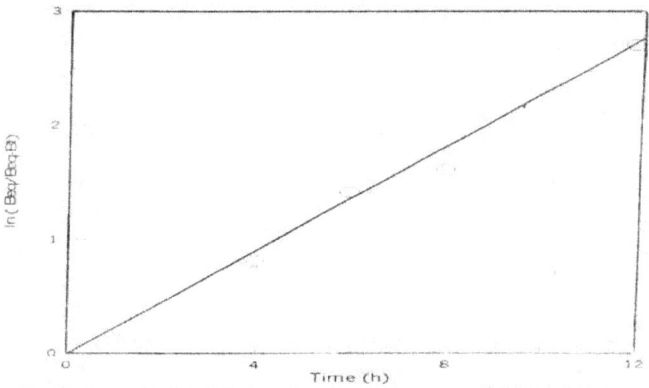

b- pseudo first order kinetic analysis of the association time course

c-first order kinetic analysis of the dissociation time course. For calculation of the dissociation rate constant, the initial more rapid component was corrected for the contribution due to the slower second component as indicated by the dashed line

Fig   Kinetics of ^{125}I-hCG binding to the purified hCG - receptor

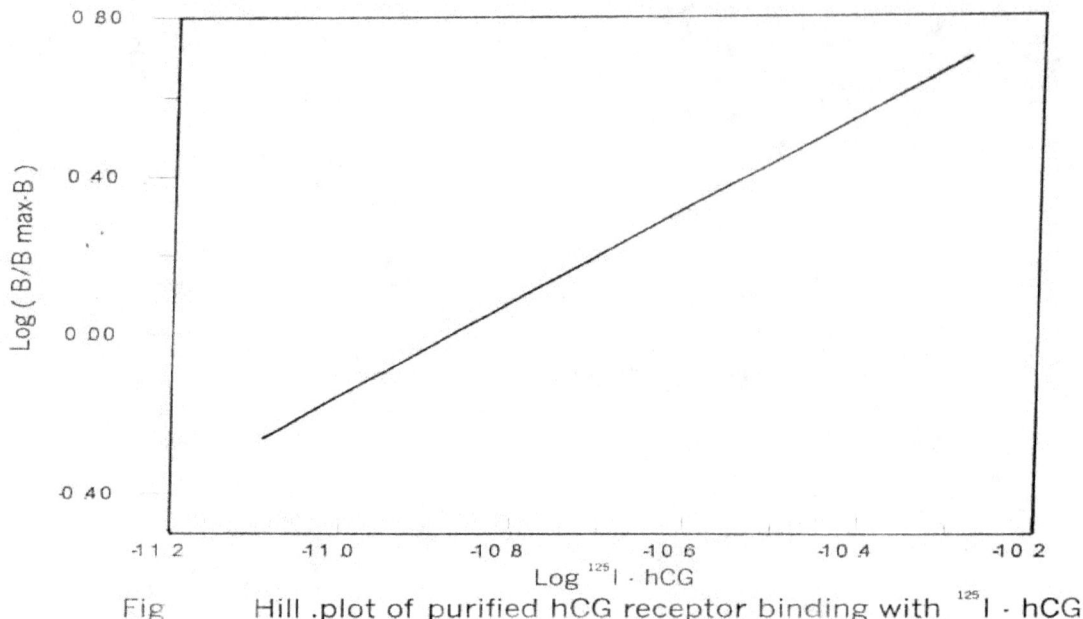

Fig   Hill .plot of purified hCG receptor binding with ^{125}I - hCG

Chapter Five

Evaluation of Some Biochemical Constituents in Gynecologic Cancers

Chapter Five

Evaluation of Some Biochemical Constituents in Gynecologic Cancers

Abstract

The levels of CEA were slightly elevated above the reference value(5ng/ml) in the sera of 33% of patients with endometrial cancer and 43% of patients with ovarian cancer..CEA immunoreactivity of malignant ovarian tissue extracts were significantly elevated than in corresponding serum samples, while it was not significantly elevated in malignant uterine tissue extracts. CEA was found in the sera of 7% of control and 11-13% of patients with benign tumors, which indicate the non specify of this tumor marker for gynecologic cancers.

The LDH activity was higher in patients with ovarian and endometrial cancers than those of healthy individuals but not statistically significant. The highest elevation of LDH activity was observed in the invasive stages. The electrophoresis analysis of LDH isoenzymes for serum of ovarian cancer showed extra band.

The total AlP activity and HSAP activity in the sera of cancer patients were significantly higher than in control group. The differences in HSAP activity between malignant and control were clear.

Copper, Zinc, and Calcium concentration were measured in the sera of the patients with ovarian and uterine cancers by flame atomic absorption spectrophometry. Zinc levels were significantly higher in cancer patients than in control group. Copper levels did not alter in cancer patients than in control. The patients with ovarian and endometrial cancer (without metastasis) showed no significant differences in their sera calcium levels from those of the control group.

Introduction:

Increased levels of several antigens, oncofetal proteins, ectopic hormones and enzymes have been considered as potential tumor markers in gynecologic cancers for helping in screening, diagnosis, staging, prognosis and monitoring of cancer therapy.

The elevation of oncofetal antigen, carcinoembryonicantigen(CEA), have been demonstrated in a large variety of cancers [249,250]. The frequency of elevated concentration varies with the tumor type and the stage of disease, generally, being higher in patients with metastasis. Serial CEA determination has been effective in predicting occult recurrence in patients whose tumor contain high antigen concentration. There are a number of reports on the clinical values of circulating CEA in patients with uterine tumor, elevated plasma level was found in 14-100% of cases of endometrial cancer[251-253]. Elevation plasma concentrations of CEA have also been found in ovarian cancer and often in mucinous histotypes[254][255][26]. Immunohistochemical studies demonstrated that CEA was higher in cervical squamous cell carcinoma tissue than in endometrial cancer[256-258], therefore it might be useful for differentiating endocervical from endometrial.

Lactate dehydrogenase (LDH) is an enzyme in the glycolytic pathway and is released as the results of cell damage. The elevation of LDH in malignancy is nonspecific. LDH has been demonstrated in a variety of cancer such as breast, colon, stomach, liver, germ cell testicular, lung cancer and Hodgkin's lymphoma[44]. The significance of increased serum LDH levels in gynecological cancers have been documented[259][43][45-47]. The serum LDH level has been shown to be correlated with tumor mass in solid tumors and provided a prognostic indicator of disease progression. The changes in activity of serum LDH isoenzymes provided some specificity for organ involvement[44][45].

Alkaline Phosphatase (ALP)enzyme may arise from liver, bone or placenta. Elevated levels of ALP are seen in primary or secondary liver cancer and prostate cancer. Its level may be helpful in evaluating metastasis cancer with bone or liver involvement. Other malignancies such as leukemia, breast, and lung cancer with bone or liver metastases also manifest elevated ALP. The heat stable alkaline phospatase (HSAP) has been designated as carcinoplacental protein following the observation that an isoenzyme of ALP biochemically and immunologically is vary similar to placental alkaline phosphatase which ectopically expressed by some cancer cells[48][260]. This isoenzyme has been measured in the sera of patients with varying degree of tumors of the cervix, corpus uteri and ovaries[49][261][262] and with Hodgkins disease[263] and breast cancer[50].

Different elements are constituents for, or interact with enzymes and hormones that regulate the metabolism of much larger amounts of biochemical substrates, affecting the permeability of cell membranes, and other mechanism[264]. Therefore it is attracted attention in cancer research. Many of the trace elements such as copper, zinc, and essential elements such as calcium have been studied in different cancers. Zinc is needed as cofactor in nucleic acid polymerases and is therefore connected to high mitotic activity of tumor cells. Thus, an elevated zinc serum levels in cancers patients might be a consequence of tumor development[265]. Serum copper levels have also be studied in different type of malignancies such as breast, lung, Kidney tumors, it appeared to be increase in some cancers and frequently return to normal levels after resection[266]. Cancer has been considered to be the commonest cause of hypercalcaemia which occurs in approximately 10-20% of patients suffering from cancer[267]. Hypercalcaemia in cancer without the presence of bone metastasis was described by the finding of the parathyroid hormone (PTH)-like peptides[268], or by a mechanism involving elevated levels of 1,25-dihydroxy vit.D3[269], or by releasing locally osteoclast activating factors which stimulate osteoclastic resorption of bone[270]. Hypercalcaemia is almost associated with squamous cell tumors and parathyroid hormone-like material was extracted from a sequamous cell lung tumors[271]

In this chapter CEA levels in sera and tissues of patients with ovarian and uterine tumors were determined by immunoradiometric assay (IRMA). The activity of LDH and ALP were measured by colorimetric methods. LDH isonenzymes were analyzed by electrophoresis. HSAP was also determined. In addition copper, zinc, and calcium concentration were determined in the sera of the ovarian and uterine tumors patients. All biochemical constituents were evaluated for their usefulness in gynecologic cancers.

Material and Methods

5.1 CEA, LDH, and AIP Kits

1- Carcinoemryonic antigen (CEA) IRMA Kit was provided by (OCPA.France) and contains one vial of ^{125}I-rabbit-antiCEA antibody, one hundred test tubes coated with anti CEA antibodies, seven vials of human CEA standard with concentrations ranging of (0-200 ng/ml), two vials of control serum, one vial of assay buffer, and tube of wash reagent.

2- Lactate dehydrogenase (LDH) Kit for colorimetric determination was provided by (Randox, England) and contains one vial of 0.8 mmol/l sodium pyruvate in phosphate buffer PH 7.45, 10 Vial of NADH (1mg/ml)(each vial content reconstituted with 10ml of buffer before used), and one vial of color reagent (1mmol/L 2,4-dinitrophenydrazine in hydrochloric acid).

3- Alkaline phosphates Kit for colorimetric determination was provided by (bio Merieux-Frane) and contains substrate buffer vial (5mmol/l Dinatriumphenylphosphate in 50 mmol/l carbonate bicarbonate buffer pH 10), standard phenol reagent equal to 20 Kind and King U, inhibitor reagent (60mmol/l amino -4antipyrine with 75 g/l sodium arsenate), color reagent (150mmol/l potassium ferricyanide).

5.2 Apparatus

The apparatus, mentioned in section 2.2 were used in the experiments of this chapter.

5.3 Patients and Specimens

The study group consisted of benign and malignant patients, and control group described in section 2.3. The sera of these groups were collected as described in section 2.4.and tissues homogenates and were prepared as described in section 2.4.

5.4 CEA Quantitative Measurement

The level of CEA was measured in the sera and tissues of patients by the immunoradiometric assay (IRMA). The assay protocol was described in Table 5.1., according to manufacturer instructions.

5.5 Determination of LDH Activity

Colorimetric method was used to determine LDH activity. The method is based on the reduction of pyruvate to lactate in the presence of NADH by the action of lactate dehydrogenase.

$$\text{Pyruvate} + NADH + H^+ \xrightarrow{\text{LDH}} \text{Lacate} + NAD^+$$

The pyruvate that remains unchanged reacts with 2,4-dinitrophenylhydrazine to give the corresponding phenylhydrazone which is determined calorimetrically in alkaline medium at 520 nm. The assay protocol was described in Table 5.2, according to manufacture instructions

Table (5.1): Assay protocol of CEA

Tube number	CEA standards ng/ml							Control serum	Samples
	0	2.3	4.8	9.6	19.6	60.0	210.0		
	1,2	3,4	5,6	7,8	9,10	11,12	13,14	15,16	17,18
Standard Control Patient samples (µL)	←-------------------------------------- 100uL --------------------------------------→								
Assay buffer (µL)	←-------------------------------------- 100 µL --------------------------------→								
	Shaking for 2h at 25 °C								
Wash buffer (ml)	←----------------------------1 ml --→ Aspirate, wash once with wash buffer								
^{125}I-anti CEA (µL)	←----------------------------100uL ----------------------------------→								
	Shaking for 1h at 25°C								
Wash buffer (ml)	←----------------------------1 ml --→								
	Aspirate, wash once with wash buffer, measurment of the radioactivity bound in gamma counter								

Calculation

1- The radioactivity of all standards measured in (CPM) bound was plotted vs. their concentration (Fig 5.1).

2- The samples and control values of CEA were read from standard curve.

Table 5.2 : Assay protocol of LDH

Tube number	Sodium pyruvate with NADH(U/L)						Serum sample
	0	111.4	223.1	334.9	390.6	446.3	
	1,2	3,4	5,6	7,8	9,10	11,12	13,14
Sodium pyruvate with NADH(ml)	0.9	0.7	0.5	0.3	0.2	0.1	0.9
Distilled water(ml)	0.1	0.3	0.5	0.7	0.8	0.9	
Serum sample(ml)							0.1
	Mixing, incubation in a water bath at 37°C for exactly 30 min							
Color reagent	←-------------------------------1 ml --------------------------------→						
	Mixing, let stand at room temperature for 20 min						
1.6% NaOH(ml)	←---------------------------10 ml --------------------------------→						
	Mixing, let stand at room temperature for 10 min. Reading absorbance of sample or standards against distilled water at 520 nm						

Calculations:

1- The absorbance of samples (1-12) are plotted vs. the corresponding values in U/L (Fig 5.2).

2- The serum LDH activity was determined from calibration curve.

5.6 Analysis of LDH by Electrophoresis

LDH isoenzyme was separated by poly acrylamide gel electrophoresis as described in section (4.6.2). The enzyme activity bands were developed according to following reactions[272]:

$$\text{Lactate} + \text{NAD}^+ \xrightarrow{\text{LDH}} \text{Pyryvate} + \text{NADH} + \text{H}$$

$$\text{NADH} + \text{Phenazain methosulfate} \longrightarrow \text{NAD}^+ + \text{Phenazin methosulfate}$$

$$\text{Phenaz methosulfate (PMS)} + \text{nitroblue tetrazolium (MBT)} \longrightarrow \text{Nitroblue tetrazolium formazan (Violt ppt)} + \text{phenazain methosulfate}$$

After electrophoresis, the working solution was added on the gel, then incubation for 60 min at 37°C, The violet bands appeared and the gel was placed in fixing solution for 10 min to fix the bands.

Solutions:

Working solution: was prepared by mixing 1ml of 2 mol/l sodium lactate, 3ml of 1mg/ml NBT, 0.3ml of 1mg/ml/PMS and 1ml of 0.056 mol/l Tris buffer pH 7.4 then 15 mg of NAD^+ was added.

Fixing solution: was prepared by mixing methanol, distilled water, glacial acetic acid in ratio of 5:4:1

5.7 Determination of Alkaline Phosphates Activity

Colorimetric method was used to determine AIP activity according to the following reaction

$$\text{Phenylphosphate} \xrightarrow{\text{Alkaline phosphatase, pH10}} \text{phenol + phosphate}$$

The liberated phenol was measured in the presence of amino 4-antipyrine and potassium ferricyanide. The presence of sodium arsenate in the reagent stops the enzymatic reaction. The assay protocol was described in Table 5.3: according to manufacturer instructions.

Table 5.3 Assay protocol of ALP

Tube number	Serum sample 1,2	Serum blank 3,4	Standard 5,6	Reagent 7,8
Substrate buffer (ml)	←----------------------------------2 ml ----------------------------------→			
	Incubation for 5 min at 37°C			
Serum sample (µL)	←--50 µl ---→			
Standard (µL)			←--50 µl ---→	
	Incubation exactly 15 min at 37°C			
Inhibitor	←----------------------------------0.5 ml ----------------------------------→			
	Mixing			
Color reagent	←----------------------------------0.5 ml ----------------------------------→			
Serum sample		←--50 µl ---→		
Distilled water				←--50 µl ---→
Mixing, let stand for 10 min in the dark. Reading absorbance at 510 nm against reagent blank				

Calculation

$A_{serum\ sample} - A_{serum\ blank} / A_{standard}$ X 142

Kind and king U/L=Enzyme activity unit=One kind and king unit is that an mount of enzyme which in the given conditions liberates 1mg of phenol in 15 min at 37°C

4.8 Determination of Heat Stable Alkaline Phosphatase Activity (HSAP):

Heat stable alkaline phosphatase (HSAP) activity was measured after the complete inactivation of all AIP isoenzymes by heating the sample for 15 min at 55°C in a water bath[50]. Fifty microliter of serum sample was incubated for 15 min at 55°C in a water bath. Immediately after incubation the inactivated serum was cooled at ice temperature. The remaining activity was measured by the same methods of AIP (section 5.7)

4.9 Determination of the Elements (Cu^{++}, Zn^{++}, Ca^{++}) Concentrations in the Sera of Tumor Patients

Copper, zinc,Ca were determined by flame atomic absorption spectorphotometry[73].Serum trace element levels were measured using serum diluted (1:2) with deionized distilled water, while Ca^{++} level was measured using serum diluted (1:10) with deionized distills water. The concentrations of the elements were determined by comparing the signal from diluted serum with that from appropriate aqueous calibration standards, which were prepared. Patients with metastases were excluded when calcium was determined.

Results and Discussion

Biochemical Constituents in Ovarian and Endometrial Cancer Patients

The levels of the biochemical constituents in the sera of patients studies were as summarized in Tables 5.4, 5.5, and 5.6. As can be seen from the Tables, all the biochemical constituents had higher mean values in patients as compared to the controls.

CEA levels of sera of ovarian and endometrial cancer patients were slightly elevated and most modestly elevated in endometrial cancer. CEA was elevated in 43% of ovarian cancer and 33% of endometrial cancer patients as compared to 7% in the control population Table (5.4). The incidence of antigen elevation in patients with invasive cancer was 25% higher than that in patients with stage I cancer. The higher levels of CEA were found in patients with mucinous ovarian neoplasms. CEA immunoreactivity also has been determined in the patient's tissues. The elevation of tissue CEA levels appeared to be statistically significant than in the corresponding sera samples ($p<0.05$) in ovarian malignant condition (Fig 5.3), while the difference was not significant in endometrial cancer. The results of determination of the CEA in the sera and tissues of gynecologic tumor patients indicated that CEA was not tumor specific and was found in some benign conditions. These results confirms previous observation from other investigator, where CEA activity in tissues can be demonstrated in most gynecological cancers while serum levels are often too modestly elevated to be useful for diagnosis or for monitoring. Stall et.al.,[255] showed slightly elevated plasma CEA level in approximately 50% of ovarian cancer patients, and mucinous tumors tend to have highest levels. Tuxen et.al., [26] also found elevated serum CEA levels in patients with mucinous histotypes ovarian cancer. Bast et.al., [39], and Tuxen et.al., [26][254] obtained that the combination of CEA and CA125 would have a higher sensitivity and specificity than CA125 alone, in monitoring human ovarian cancer. In the uterus, adenocarcinoma that arise in the endocervix express a greater amount of CEA than adenocarcinomas of the endometriums [251-253]. It is reflected in the reported frequency of elevated plasma CEA level: 68% in cervical adenocarcinoma and 34% in endometrial adenocarcinoma, therefore, have therapeutic consequences when doubt exists as to the origin of a uterine tumor[40]. Squamous cell carcinoma of cervical cancers also express CEA and high levels indicated in advanced disease[41]. In immunohistochemical studies, CEA was detected in 60-63% of cervical squamous cell carcinoma, and in 77% of cases of cervical adenocarcinoma [256-258]. Generally, in gynecologic cancers a high pretreatment values of serum CEA indicate awide spread of tumor[99] and poor prognosis[251-253]. CEA have also been demonstrated in a large variety of malignancies included, cancers of the colon and pancreas and elevated concentration, varies with the tumor type and the stage of disease [249][250]. CEA also elevated in several non cancerous condition, such as smoking or hepatic dysfunction.

It is evident from the Table 5.5 that the mean levels of LDH activity were higher in cancer patients then those of healthy individuals but the differences were not statistically significant. The highest elevation of LDH activity was observed the invasive stage of ovarian cancer (stage I FIGO.133±24.343 U/L, and satageII+III

FIGO.185.6±47.54U/L). The electrophoresis pattern of serum LDH isoenzyme in ovarian cancers (Fig 5.4) showed an additional band (extra band). This extra isoenzyme moved faster than LDH_1 which means that its charge is more negative than LDH_1. LDH, is elevated in the sera of patients with a variety of cancers[259]. Evaluation of serum levels of this enzyme was documented to be significantly advantageous in diagnosis and treatment monitoring of patients with gynecological cancers[43-47], and its level reflect tumor burden as well as tumor growth or regression .However LDH as single marker has not proved sufficient to meet the full requirements of clinical application. Increased serum LDH value in malignancies is multifunctional and no single explanation can be put forward of account for whole spectrum of malignancies. LDH is often elevated in epithelial ovarian cancer[259], cervical cancer[47] and many solid malignancies[17], making it a non-specific tumor marker. This isoenzyme provide marginal specificity for organ involvement[44]. The elevation of LDH_5 was associated with liver metastases and central nervous system metastases[17]. In dysgerminom, the two fast fraction(s)(LDH_1 and LDH_2) were increased and their activity appeared to parallel the response to therapy[45], LDH_3 was found to be elevated in multiple myeloma. Add ional band has been found in hepato cellular cancer patients[17].

The results of total AIP determination indicated that the mean values in cancer patients were higher than control and significantly different (Table 5.6). Different stages of ovarian and endometrial cancers appeared different levels of total AIP. The results of HSAP estimation showed that mean value in patients with ovarian and endometrial cancers were significantly increase compared to the control group (Table 5.6).

The HSAP levels did not correlate with tumor stage. This isoenzyme has been found to be more useful as tumor marker in gynecologic cancers than total AIP because the differences between cancer and control groups were clear. It has been reported that HSAP appeared in 21-22% of cases of cervical cancer and in 25% of cases of endometrial cancer[260][261]. Elevated serum HSAP has been found in 64% of ovarian cancer patients[49], but by using a radioimmunoassay and a polyclonal antibody for placental AIP determination, only 18% of cases showed elevated levels .HSAP has previously been reported to be useful in combination with lipid bound sialic acid (LSA), in diagnosis, and treatment monitoring for cancer patients [50][274]. The changes in the HSAP level were also reported in benign tumor of ovary[49][261].

Copper, Zinc, Calcium in the Sera of Ovarian and Endometrial Cancer Patients

The results of determination copper, zinc, and calcium ions concentration are illustrated in Table (5-7). These results showed that sera zinc levels were significantly higher ($p<0.05$) in ovarian and endometrial cancers groups than in the control group. In benign group, zinc levels remained without alteration .Serum copper levels were not significantly higher in the two cancer groups when compared with those of controls, although the mean values were higher in cancers groups. No alteration in the level of copper ion was observed in the sera of benign tumor as compared to healthy individual. The patients with ovarian and endometrial cancers showed no significant difference in their sera calcium levels from those of the control group. However, two patients of ovarian cancer and one of endometrial cancers were hypercalcemic (10.5, 11.1 and 10.6 mg/dl respectively).

High levels of zinc in the ovarian and endometrial cancer are in agreement with studies that indicate, the zinc level was increased in different cancer patients[275][265][261]. It has been suggested that the zinc might play a possible role in tumor growth promotion.

The copper in serum exists largely in the form of ceruloplasmin (more than 90%) a metalloprotein of Mwt (132 kDa) contain 6 atoms of copper/ molecule[275].

The copper levels of cancer sera in our study did not significantly change but some studies reported elevation in ceruloplasmin level in some cancer such as breast and lung cancers[256]. It is known that copper plays some role in angiogenesis, where it is required for development of new tissue as well as tumor growth possibly through the mediation of copper –dependent amine oxidases. The increase of zinc to copper ratio in the sera of cancer patients reflects the implication of the zinc and copper in the cancerous process of the tissue, so it may be useful as a tumor marker for the evaluation of the status of gynecologic cancers.

Although the mean values in the present study for ovarian and endometrial cancers patients showed no significant difference in their sera calcium levels, from those of the control group, but some cancer patients were hypercalcaemic. Hypercalcemia is a common complication of cancer and usually associated with bone metastasis[270]. Calcium is present in serum in three distinct fractions, free or ionized calcium account for about 50% of total calcium, about 5% complexed with variety of anions particularly phosphate and citrate, and the remaining 45% of Ca is bound to plasma protein especially to albumin[276]. Calcium homeostasis involves three major organs, the small intestine, the kidney and the skeleton. Hypercalcemia has been reported in breast, lung, kidney cancers without the presence of bone metastases[268]. PTH like peptides were found in about 49% of patients with malignant hypercalcaemia and 16% of patients with malignant normocalcaemic state. It have also been reported that cancer tissue in the human being was capable of direct osteolysis[277]. Rieke et.al.,[269] reported a hypercalcemic state (with the absence of bone destruction) in Hodgkins disease. They suggested elevated levels of 1,25 dihydroxy Vit D3. Hypercalcamia on malignancy was thought to be due to progression of the tumor tissue[277]. Hypercalcacmia has also referred to osteoclast activating factors which are released locally by tumor. These include prostaglandin E2[278], interlukin I, tumor necrosis factor[279] such as Beta lymphotoxin, epidermal growth factor [280], and transforming growth factor beta[281].

Table 5.4 The values of CEA levels in sera of patients with gynecologic tumors

(All details are explained in the text)

Tumor	Group	%of elevated CEA >5ng/ml *(Elevated /total)	Mean ± S.E.M of all patients ng/ml	Statistical *significant
Ovarian	*C	7(2/30)	3.96±1.25	
	*B	11(4/35)	4.11±1.79	*NS
	*M	43(6/14)	12.25±12.8	P<0.05
Uterine	C	7(2/30)	3.96±1.25	
	B	13(3/24)	3.97±1.76	NS
	M	33(3/9)	6.33±3.64	P<0.05

*C: control

*B: benign

*M: malignant

NS: not significant

Elevated/Total:numberof patients with CEA above 5mg/ml/number of patients with CEA below 5mg/ml.

Table 5.5 Lactate dehydrogenase (LDH) activity in sera of patients with gynecologic tumors (All details are explained in the text)

Tumor	Group	*N	mean±S.E.M(U/ml)	Statistical significance
Ovarian	*C	30	144.78±32.5	
	*B	35	145.6±24.7	NS
	*M	14	156.57±28.8	NS
Uterine	C	30	144.78±30.5	
	B	24	143.93±26.5	NS
	M	9	146.51±67.34	NS

C:control

B:benign

M:malignant

NS:not significant

N:number of patients.

Table 5.6 AIP activity and HSAP activity in sera of patients with gynecologic tumors (All details are explained in the text)

T tumor	Group	*N	mean ±S.E.M of AIP U/L	Statistical significance	mean ±S.E.M. of HSAP U/L	Statistical significance
Ovarian	C	30	58.5±19.4		2.3±0.3	
	B	35	60.3±12.3	NS	2.2±0.6	NS
	M	14	81.5±26.5	P<0.05	5.5±0.4	P<0.05
Uterine	C	30	58.5±19.4		2.3±0.3	
	B	24	65.9±14.6	NS	2.4±0.9	NS
	M	9	78.5±32.3	P<0.05	4.6±0.5	P<0.05

*M: Malignant

*B: Benign

* C control

*N: Number of patients

*NS: Not Significant

Table 5.7 Copper (Cu^{++}), Zinc (Zn^{++}) and Calcium (Ca^{++}) concentration in the sera of ovarian and endometrial cancers patients

Tumor	No. of patients	Copper mean±S.E.M µmol/l	Zinc mean± µmol/l	Zn^{++}/Cu^{++}	Calcium men±S.E.mg/100ml
Ovarian *M *B *C	8 10 25	17.3±1.5 16.6±1.6 16.7± 0.71	13.3±3.2 7.4±1.1 7.1 ± 0.45	0.75 0.44 0.42	10.1±1.2 9.5±0.08 9.7 ± 0.7
Uterine *M *B *C	9 10 25	17.4±1.8 17.1± 0.85 16.7± 0.71	10.7 ± 2.15 6.8 ± 1.9 7.1 ± 0.45	0.61 0.4 0.42	9.9±0.3 9.6±0.16 9.7±0.7

*M: Malignant

*B: Benign

*C: Control

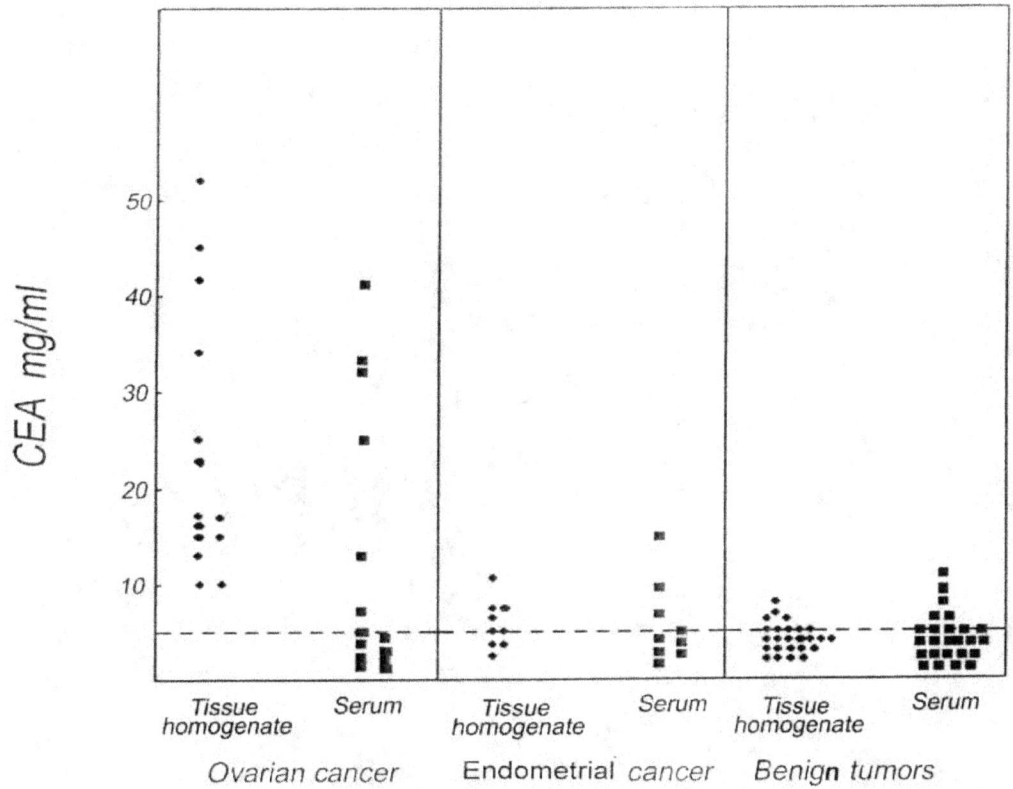

Fig   Distribution of the individual levels of the CEA (ng/ml) in the sera and tissues homogentes of benign and malignant gynecologic tumors

Fig. Electrophoresis pattern of serum LDH isonzymes of ovarian cancer patient
1, 2: control
3, 4: benign
5, 6: malignancy

Conclusions :

1- Determination of total serum intact hCG and free hCGβ or free hCGβ is of great clinical diagnostic value for ovarian and endometrial cancers than determination of only intact hCG.

2- Determination of intact hCG and free hCG in malignant tissues found to be of diagnostic value for gynecologic cancers.

3- The developed protocol for the assay of hCG-Rs is capable to analyze these receptor and the procedure is suitable for the assessment of such receptors in benign and malignant gynecologic tumors.

4- Purification of hCG receptor from ovarian cancer indicated that this receptor is functional in malignant conditions.

5- Determination of CEA immunoreactivities in cancer tissues may be useful for differentiating between gynecologic cancer.

6- LDH enzyme activity can be used for the assessment of the aggressiveness gynecologic cancers. Also LDH isoenzymes analysis may be useful for diagnostic these cancers, where it had been showed extra band different from normal serum.

7- HSAP isoenzyme could be used for the diagnostic of gynecologic cancer better than total ALP activity.

8- Serum Zinc to Copper ratio may be introduced as a biochemical marker in the diagnosis of gynecologic cancers.

The Future Work

According to the results obtained in this thesis, the flowing works are suggested for the future :

1- Investigation the free hCGβ subunit in more cases, and more type of gynecologic cancers such as cancer of cervix, vagina, and vulva .

2- Studies the expression of hCG and its subunits on the cell membrane of cultured human cancer cells using flow cytometric technique.

3- Preparation of monoclonal antibodies for free hCGβ subunit and for hCG-Rs to use them for hCG and its receptor identity as diagnostic tools for tumor .

4- Isolation of the m-RNAs encoding hCG-Rs and cloning the cDNA of these receptors , then comparison the purified receptors obtained in this study with those produced by the cDNA technology to elucidate the actual native species of hCG-R within the ovarian tumor.

5- Evaluation of the anti-hCG vaccine, which used for the prevention of pregnancy to prevent cancer. The studies must be including the adjuvant application of anti-hCG vaccines for the diagnosis and treatment of patients with cancer.

References:

1. Berek J.S., Hacker N.F. eds. **Practical Gynecologic Oncology.** 3rd ed. Philadelphia: Lippincott Williams & Wilkins, 2000.
2. **Results of IRAQI Cancer Registry.** (a):1992-1994,(b)1995 -1997. Cancer board Minsitry of health .IRAQI Baghdad; 1996 (a) , 1999 (b).
3. Eisner R. P. and Berek J.S. **Gynecologic Cancers**. In Dennis A., Casiato M.D. , Barry B. and Lowirz M.D. (eds) Manual of Clinical Oncology 4th ed. Philadelphia:lippincott Williams & Wilkins, 2000, P238-268.
4. Parazzini F. , Vecchia C.L. , Bocciolone L. and Franceschi S. 1991. **The Epidemiology of Endometrial Cancer (Review)**. Gynecol . Oncol. 410:1-16.
5. Seiden M.V. 2001 **Ovarian Cancer**. The Oncologist 6:327-332.
6. Burke T.W., Luna G. T., Malpica A. Baker V.V. Whittaker L. and Mitchell M.F. 1996 **Endometrial Hyperplasia and Endometrial Cancer.** Gynecol Cancer prevention 23:411-456.
7. Ambros R.A., Ballouk F. Malfetano J.H. et.al. 1994 **Significance of Papillary (Villoglandular) Differentiation in Endometrioid Carcinoma** Am. J.Surg. Pathol .18:569-574.
8. Brinton L.A., Berman M.L., Mortel R., et.al. 1992 **Reproductive , Menstrual and Medical Risk Factors for Endometrial Cancer** Am. J. Obstet. Gynecol .167:1317-1322.
9. Allan J. **Ovarian Cancer.** Clinical Symposia (Vol 48) New Jersey:Ciba-Geigy Corporation 1996.
10. Alper O., DeSantis M.L. Stambery K. et.al. 2000 **Antisense Suppression of Epidermal Growth Factor Receptor Expression Alters Cellular Proliferation, Cell-adhesion , and Tumorigenicity in Ovarian Cancer Cell.** Int. J. Cancer. 88:566-574.
11. Rosal J. ed. **Ackermans Surgical pathology** 8th ed. St. Louis (U.S.A): Mosby year book, 1996, p1461.
12. Tait DI, Thigpen JT. **Advances in Gynecologic Cancer Program and Abstracts of the 37th Annual Meting of the American Society of Clinical Oncology**, San Francesico, California, May 12-15, 2001.
13. Vasey P.A. Atkinson R., Coleman R. et. al. 2001 **Docetaxel- carboplatin as first line chemotherapy for Epithtial Ovarian Cancer.** Br. J. Cancer 84:170-178.
14. Markman M. Kennedy A., Webster K.,et al. 2001 **Combination Chemotherapy with Carboplatin and Docetaxelin in the Treatment of Cancer of the Ovary and Fallopian Tube and Primary Carcinoma of the Peritoneum.** J. Clin Oncol. 19:1901-1905.
15. Williams C.J. 1998 **Tamoxifen in Relapsed Ovarian Cancer: a systematic review** .Int. J. Gyncol Cancer 8:89-94.
16. Markman M., Bookman M.A., 2000 **Second- line Treatment of Ovarian Cancer**. The Oncologist 5:26-35.
17. Onsrud M. 1991 **Tumor Markers in Gynecologic Oncology**. Scand J Clin Lab Invest. Suppl 206:60-70.
18. Daunter B. 1990 **Tumor Markers in Gynecologic Oncology** (Review) Gynecol. Oncol. 39:1-15.
19. Rademacher T.W., Parekh R.B., and Dwek R.A. 1988 **Glycobiology** Ann. Rev .Biochem. 57:785-838.
20. Kato H.,TorigoeT. 1997 **Radioimmunoassay for Tumor Antigen of Human Cervical Squamous Cell Carcinoma**. Cancer 40:1621-1624.

21- Senikjian E.K., Young J.M., Weiser P.A. 1987 **An Evaluation of Squamous Cell Carcinoma Antigen in Patient with Cervical Squamous Cell Carcinoma** Am J Obstet Gynecol. 157:433-437.
22- Scambia G., Panici P.B., Baiocchi G., et.al. 1991 **The Value of Sequamous cell Carcinoma Antigen in Patients with locally Advanced Cervical Cancer Undergoing Neadjuvant Chemotherapy**. Am J obsret Gynecol 164:631-634.
23- Bast B. J., Klug T. L., St John E., et al. 1983 **A Radioimmunoassay Using Monoclonal Antibody to Monitor the Course of Epithelial Ovarian Cancer**. N Engl J Med. 309:883-887.
24- Bon G., Kenemans P., Verstraeten R. , Van Kamp G., and Hilgers J. 1996 **Serum Tumor Marker Immunoassays in Gynecologic Oncology: Establishment of references values**. Am J Obstet Gynecol 174:107-114.
25- Tuxen M.K., Soletormos G., Dombernowsky G. 1995 **Tumor Markers in the Management of Patients with Ovarian Cancer.** Cancer Treat. Rev. 21:215-245.
26- Tuxen M.K., Soletormos G., Petersen P., Schioler V., and Dombernowsky G.,1999 **Assessment of Biological Variation and Analytical Imprecision of CA.125, CEA, and TPA in Relation to Monitoring of Ovarian Cancer.** Gynecol Oncol. 74:12-22.
27- Niloff J.M., Klug A., Schaetzl E., et.al. 1984 **Elevation of Serum CA.125 in Carcinoma of the Fallopian Tube, Endometrium, and Endocervix.** Am J Obsret Gynecol 148:1057-1059.
28- Abrao M.S., Podgaec S., Filho B.M. , Ramos L.O., Pinotti J.A. , and Oliveira R.M. 1997 **The use of Biochemical Markers in the Diagnosis of Pelvic Endometriosis.** Human Reproduction 12:2523-2527.
29- Buamah P.K.,,,, Skillen A.W. 1994 **Serum CA.125 Concentration in Patients with Benign Ovarian Tumors.** J. Surg Oncol 56:71-74.
30- Jacobs I.J., Fay T.W., Lower A.M. 1989. **The London Hospital Ovarian Cancer Screening Project**. Proc 2nd meeting Int. Gynecol Cancer Soc, Toronto :167.
31- Onsurd M., Vergoto I., Moen M. 1988 **CA-125 in Peritoneal Fluids of Healthy Women and of Patients with Ovarian Carcinoma** .Proc 24th meeting Scand Soc Obstet Gynecol ,Trondheim:49.
32- Koprowski H., Steplewski Z., Mitchell K., et.al. 1979 **Colorectal Carcinoma Antigens Detected by Hybridoma Antibodies.** Somatic Cell Genet 5:957-961.
33- Hilkens J., Bulis F., Hilgers J, et.al. 1984 **Monoclonal Antibodies Against Human Milk–fat Globule Membranes Detection Deferential Antigens of the Mammary Gland and its tumor.** Int J. Cancer 34:197-200.
34- Scambia G., Benedetti P., Baiocchi G., et.al. 1988 **CA 15-3 as aTumor Marker in Gynecological Malignancies.** Gynecol Oncol 30:265-273.
35- Bon G., Keneman P., Vankamp G.J. Yedema C.A., and Hilgers J 1990 **Review on the Clinical Value of Polymorphic Epithelial Mucin Tumor Marker for the Management of Carcinoma Patients.** Nucl Med Allied Sci. 34:151-162.
36- Yedema C., Kenemans P., Wobbes T., 1991 **Carcinoma –Associated Mucin Serum Marker CA M26 and CA M29: efficacy in detecting and monitoring patients with caner of the breast,colon,ovary, endometrium and cervix.** Int J. Cancer 47:170-179.
37- Knauf S. 1988 **Clinical Evaluation of Ovarian Tumor NB/70K: monoclonal antibody assays for distinguishing ovarian cancer from other gynecologic disease.** Am J Obstet. Gynecol. 158:1067-1071.

38- Petru E., Sevin B., Averette H.E., 1990 **Comparison of Three Tumor Markers –CA-125, Lipid associated Scialic Acid (LSA), and NB /70K. in Monitoring Ovarian Cancer**. Gynecol Oncol.38:181-185.
39- Bast R.C., Klug T.L., Schaetzl E., et. al. 1984 **Monitor Human Ovarian Carcinoma with a Combination of CA-125, CA 19-9 and a CEA**. Am J. Obstet Gynecol 149:553-558.
40- KjQrstad K.E., Rjaster H. 1977 **Studies on Carcinoembryonic Antigen level in Patients with Adenocarcinoma of the Uterus**. Cancer 40:2953-55.
41- KjQrstad K.E., Rjaster H. 1977 **Carcinoembryonic Antigen levels in Patients with Squamous cell Carcinoma**. Obstet Gynocol 51:293-296.
42- Genest D., Sheets E., Lage J., et.al. 1994 **Flow Cytometric Analysis of Nuclear DNA Content in Endometrial Adenocarcinoma .A Typical Mitoses are Associated with DNA Aneuploidy**. Am J. Clin pathol 102:341-346.
43- Bishop A.J. , and Schiestl R.H.,2001. **Homologous Recombination as a Mechanism of Carcinogenesis**. Biochimica et. Biophysical Acta 1471:109-121.
44- Jones M.H, Koi S. and Fujimota I 1994 **Allelotype of the uterine Cancer by Analysis of RFLP and Microsatellite Polymorphisms :frequent loss of heterozygosis on chromosome** 3P, 9q, 10q, and 17P, Gene Chromosome cancer 9: 119-125.
45- Kacinski B.M., Carter D., Mittal K. et al. 1988 **High level of Expression of fms Proto-oncogene mRNA is Observed in Clinically Aggressive Human Endometrial AdenoCarcinoma** Int J. Radiat Oncol Biol Phys. 15:823-826.
46- Baiocchi G., Kavanagh J., Talpaz M, et.al. 1991 **Expression of the Macrophage Colon- Stimulating factor and its Receptor in Gynecologic Malignancies**. Cancer 67:990-996.
47- Urban J.L. 1999 **Oncogenes, Cancer and Imaging** J. Nuclear M. 40:498-504.
48- Takai N., Miyazaki T., Fuijsawa K., et.al.2001 **Expression of Polo-like Kinase in Ovarian Caner is Associated with Histological Grade and clinical Stage**. Caner letters 164:41-49.
49- Warburg O. 1956. **On the Origin of Cancer Cells Science** 123:309-314.
50- Gerorge M.A. 1978 **Carcinoma of the Ovary and Serum Lactic Dehydrogenase levels** Surg Gynecol Obstet 146:893-896.
51- Wood D.C. , Verla V., Plamqist M., and Weber F., 1973 **Serum Lactic Dehydrogenase and Isoenzyme Change in Clinical Cancer** J. Surg Oncol. 5:251-257.
52- Fujii S., Koniski I., Suzuki A.1985 **Analysis of Serum Lactic Dehydrogenase Levels and Its Isoenzymes in Ovarian Dysgerminoma** .Gynecol Oncol .22:65-68.
53- Das H.K.,Chakravorty M., and Sanyal B. 1985 **Serum Enzymes as Biochemical Markers in the Diagnosis and Prognosis of Carcinoma of the Cervix Uteri**. Ind J. Cancer 22:121-131.
54- Patel P.S. , Rawal G.N., Balar B.D. 1993 **Importance of serum Sialic Acid and lactate Dehydrogenase in Diagnosis and Treatment Monitoring of Cervical Cancer Patients**. Gynecol. Oncol 50:294-299.
55- Fishman W.H. Inglis N.R. , Green Setal . 1968 **Immunology and Biochemical of Regan Isoenzyme of Alkaline Phoshatase in Human Cancer**. Nature 219:697-700.
56- Vergote I. Onsrud M., and Nustad K. 1987 **Placental Alkaline Phoshatase as a Tumor Marker in Ovarian Cancer** . Obstet Gynecol 69:228-231.

57- Patel P.S. , Baxi B. R., Adhvaryn S. G. , and Balar D.B. 1990. **Evaluation of Serum Sialic Acid , Heat stable Alkaline phosphatase and Fucose as Markers of Breast carcinoma** . Anti Cancer Res. 10:1071-1074.
58- Lappohn R. , Burger H., Krans M. 1991. **Inhibin as a Marker for Gronulosa Cell Tumor**, Proc Symposium Scand Soc Gyncol Oncol, Gothenburg.
59- Hirose T. 1920 **Exogenous Stimulation of Corpus Luteum Formation in the Rabbit; Influence of Extracts of Human Placenta, Decidua, Fetus Hydaditimole and Corpus Luteum on the Rabbit Gonad.**J. Jpn Gynecol Soc 16:1055.
60- Ashheim S. and Zondek B. 1928 **Die Schwangerschafsdiagnose ausdem Harn durch Nachwies des Hyprophysenvorderlappen – hormone. Praktishe und theoretische Ergebnisse aus den harnuntersuchungen** .klin wochenschr 7:1453-1457.
61- Pierce J.C., and Parsons T.F. **1981 Glycoprotein hormones:Structure and Function.** Annu. Rev. BiO chem. 50:465-495.
62- Hoermann R, Spoettl G, Moncay O.R, Mann k. 1990 **Evidence for the presence of human Chorionic Gonadotropin (hCG) and Free ß-subunit of hCG in the Human Pituitary.** J.Clin Endocrinol Metab 71:179-186.
63- Jameson J.L. and Hollenberg A.N. 1993 **Regulation of Chorionic Goandotropine Gene Expression.** Endocr Rev.14:203-221.
64- Bellet D., Lazer V., Bieche I., Paradis V. , et. al 1997 **Malignant Transformation of Nontrophoblastic Cells is Associated with the Expression of Chorionic Gonadotropin ßGenes Normally Transcribed in Trophoblastic Cells** .Cancer Res. 57:516-523.
65- Ryan R.J., Charlesworth C., Mc Cormick D.J. et.al. 1988 **The Glycoprotein Hormones Recent Studies of Structure Functions Relationship** FASEB J. 2:2661-2669.
66- O'conner J. F., Birken S., Lustbader J.W., et al 1994 **Recent Advances in the Chemistry and Immunochemistry of Human Chorionic Gonadotropin. Impact on Clinical Measurement.** Endocrine Reviews 15:650-683.
67- Carlsen R.B., Bahl O.P. Swaminathan N., 1973 **Human Chorionic Gonadotropin liner Amino Acid Sequence of the ß Subunit** J. Biol Chem.. 248:6810-6827.
68- Bellisario R., Carlsen R.B., and Bahl O.P. 1973 **Human Chorionic Gonodotropin linear Amino Acid Sequence of the Alfa subunit**. J. Biol Chem. 248:6796-6809.
69- Nisula B., Connor J. 1993 **Standardization of Protein Immunoprocedures choriogonadotropin (CG)**. Scand J. Clin Lab Invest .53 (Suppl 216):42-78.
70- Thotakura N.R. Weintraub B.D., and Bahl O.P. 1990 **The Role of Carbohydrates in Human Choriogonadotropin (hCG) Action Effects of N-Linked Carbohydrate chains from hCG and other Glycoproteins on Hormonal Activity**. Molecular and Cellular Endocrinology 70:263-272.
71- Shao K. Balasubramanian S.V., Pope C.M. Bahl O.P. 1998 **Effect of Individual N-Glycosyl Chains in the ß-Subunit on the Conformation of Human Choriogonadotropin**. Molecular and Cellular Endocrinology .146:39-48.
72- Lustbader J. W., Yarmush D.L. Birken S., et.al. 1993 **The Application of Chemical Studies of Human Chorionic Gonadotropin to Visualize its Three Dimensional Structure.** Encoder.Rev 14:291-311.
73- Moyle W.R., Matzuk. M. M., Campbell P.K. et.al.1990 **Localization of Residues that confer Antibody Specificity Using Human Chorionic**

Gonadotropin Luteinizing Hormone ß-subunit Chimera and Mutants J. Biol Chem. 265:8511-8518.

74- Berger P. Bidart J.M., Delves P.S., Dirnhofer S., et.al. 1996 **Immunochemical Mapping of Gonadotropins**. Molecular and cellular Endocrinology 125:33-43.

75- Shao K., Purohil S., Bahl O.P 1996 **Effect of Modification of all loop Regions in α and ß- subunits of human Choriogonadotropin on its signal Transduction Activity**. Molecular and Cellular Endocrinology 122:173-182.

76- Wu H., Lustbader J.W., Liu Y., Canfield R.E., and Hendrickson W.A., 1994 **Structure of Human Chorionic Gonadtropin at 2.6 A° Resolution from MAD Analysis of the Selenomethionly Protein**. Structure 2:545-558.

77- Lapthorn A.J. Harris D.C. Littejohn A., Lustbader J.W., et.al. 1994 **Crystal Structure of Human Chorionic Gonadotropin**. Nature 369:455-461.

78- Lobel L. Pollak S., Wang S. Chancy M., and Lustbader J.W., 1999 **Expression and Characterization of recombinant beta subunit hCG Homodimer**. Endocrinology 10:261-70.

79- Bidart J. M.,and Bellet D. 1993 **Human Chorionic Gonadotropin Molecular Forms, Detection, and Clinical Implications Trends**. Endocrinol Metab. 4:285-291.

80- Odell W.D., Griffin J., Sawitzke A., 1990 **Chorionic Gonadotropin Secretion in Normal Nonpregnent Humans**. Trends Endocrinol Metab. 1:418-421.

81- Alfthan H., Haglund C., Dabek J. ,Stenman U.H. 1992 **Concentration of Human Choriogondotropin, Its ß-subunit, and the Core fragment of the ß-Subunit in Serum and Urine of men and nonpregnant women**. Clin chem 38:1981-1987.

82- Cole L.H. 1997 **Immunoassay of hCG, Its Free Subunits and Metabolites**. Clin chem. 43:2233-2243.

83- Skarulis M., Wehmann R.E. Nisula B.C., and Blithe D.L. 1992 **Glyecosylation Changes in Human Chorionic Gonadotropin and Free α Subunit as Gestation Progresses**. J. clin Endocrinol Metab.75:91-96.

84- Cole L.A., Tanaka A., K.m G.S., Park S-Y, et.al.1996 **Beta Core Fragment (ß -core/UGF/UGP) a Tumor Marker :seven year report**. Gynecol Oncol. 60:264-270.

85- Cole L.A. , Kadana A., Park S-Y., and Braunseten 1993 **The Deactivation of the hCG by Nicking and Dissociation**. J. Clin Endocrinol Metao 76:704-710.

86- Kardana A., Cole L.A., 1994 **Human Chorionic Gonadotropin ß-Subunit Nicking Enzymes in Pregnancy and Cancer patients serum** J. Clin Endocrinol Metab 79:761-767.

87- Birken S., Krichevsky A., O'Connor., SchlattererJ., et.al. 1999 **Development and characterization of Antibodies to a Nicked and Hyperglycosylated Form of hCG from a Choriocarcinoma patient**. Endocrine J. 7:15-24.

88- Ichikawa N.Zhai Y.L.,Shio zawa T.,Koki T.,Nogchi H., Nikaido T., Fujii S.2001 **Immunohistochemical Analysis of Cell Cycle Regulation Gene Production in Normal Trophoblast and Trophoblastic Tumor**. Int. J.Gynecol. Pathol 17:235-240.

89- Nilson J.H., Bokar J.A.,Clay C.M., Farmeric T.A., et.al. 1991 **Different Combination of Regulatory Elements may Explain Why Placenta – Specific Expression of the Glycoprotein Hormone α-Subunit Gene Occurs Only in Primates and Horses** .Biol Reprod 44:231-237.

90- Spencer K., Coombes E.J., Mallard A.S., and Ward A.M. 1992 **Free Beta Human Choriogonadotropin in Down's Syndrome Screening :a Multicentre Study of its Markers** .Ann Clin Bio Chem. 29:506-518.

91- Cole L.A., Shahabi., Rinne K.M., et.al. 1999 **Urinary Screening Tests for Fetal Down Syndrome Hyperglycosylated hCG**. Prenat Diagn 15:24-30.

92- Nishimura R., Koizume T., Yokotani T., et.al.1998 **Molecular Heterogeneity of hCG-Related Glycoprotiens and the Clinical Relevance in Trophoblastic and Nontrophoblastic Tumors** Int., J. Gynecol Obstel., 60 (Suppl 1):529-532.

93- Zon R.T., Nichol C.,Einhorn L.H. 1998 **Management Strategies and Outcomes of Germ Cell Tumor Patients with Very High Human Chorionic Gonadotrophin Levels** J.Clin Oncol 16:1294-297.

94- Elliott M., Kardana A., Lustbader J., Cole L.1997 **Carbohydrate and Peptide Structure of the Alpha –and Beta –subunits of hCG from Normal and Aberrant Pregnancy and Choriocarcinoma**. Endocrine 7:15-32.

95- Gregory J.J, and Finlay J.L 1999 **Alpha –Fetoprotein and Beta –Human Chorionic Gonadotropin: their clinical significance as tumor markers.** Drugs 57: 463-467.

96- Suzuki K., Nakazalo H., Kurokava K. Suzaki T., and Yamanaka H.1999 **Treatment of stage I Seminoma:should beta hCG Positive Seminoma be Treated Aggressively**. In. urol. Nephrol 30:593-598.

97- Rutanen E.M.And Seppala M.1978 **The hCG-Beta Subunit Radioimmunoassay In Nontrophoblastic Gynecologic Tumors.** Cancer 41:692-696.

98- Tormey D.G. Waalkes T.P., and Simon R.M. 1977 **Biological Markers in Breast Carcinoma II Clinical Correlation with Human Chorionic gonadotrophin**. Cancer 39:2391-2396.

99- Donaldson E.S., Van Nagell J.R. , Pursell S., Gay E.C., Meeker W.R, Kashmiri R. and Voorde J. 1980 **Multiple Biochemical Markers in Patients with Gynecologic Malignancies.** Cancer 45:948-953.

100- Mc Manus L.M., Naughton M.A. and Martinez H.A. 1976 **Human Chorionic Gonadotrophin in Human Neoplastic Cells.** Cancer Res. 36:3476-3481.

101- Sheth N.A., Adil M.A., Nadkarni J.J., Rajpal R. M., and Sheth A.R. 1980 **Inappropriate Secretion of Placental Lactogen and β Subunit of Human Chorionic Gonadotrophin by Cancer of the Uterine Cervix.** Gynecol oncol. 11:321-329.

102- Birkenfeld S., Noiman G., Krispin M., Schwarz S. and Zakut H. 1989 **The Incidence and Significance of Serum hCG and CEA in Patients with Gastrointestinal Malignant Disease.** Eur .J. surg. On col. 15:103-108.

103- Marcilliac I., Troalen F., Bidart J.M.,Ghillami P.,Ribrag V., Escudier B., Malassagne B. et al 1992 **Free Human Chorionic Gonadotropin βSubunit in Gonadal and Nongonadal Neoplasms.** Cancer Res. 52:3901 – 3907.

104- Alfthan H., Haglund C. Roberts P., and Stenman U.H. 1992 b. **Elevation of Free β subunit of Human Choriogonadotropin and Core β Fragment of Human choriogonadtropin in the serum and urine of Patients with Malignant Pancreatic and Biliary Disease**. cancer Res. 52:4628-4633.

105- Iles R.K., Jenkins B.J. Oliver R.T. Blandy J.P., and Chard T. 1989 **ß Human Chorionicgonadatrophin in Serum and Urine. A Marker for Metastatic Urothelial Cancer.** Br J urol 64:241-244.

106- Hoermann R.,Gerbes A.L., Spoettl G., Jungst D., and Mann K. 1992 **Immunoreactive Human Chorionic Gonadotropin and Its Free β Subunit in Serum and Ascits of Patients with Tumors.** cancer Res. 52:1520-1524.

107- Grossmann M., Hoermann R.,Gocze P.M., Ott M.,Berger P., and Mann K. 1995 **Measurement of Human Chorionic Gonadotropin Related Immunoreactivity in Serum, Acites ,and Tumor Cysts of Patients with Gynecologic Malignancies** .Eur J. clin Inv. 25:867-873.

108- Ind T., Iles R.K., Shepherd J., and Chard T., 1998 **Serum Concentration of Cancer Antigen 125, Placental Alkaline Phophatase, Cancer Associated Serum Antigen and Free Beta Human Chorionic Gonadotrophin as Prognostic Markers for Epithelial Ovarian Cancer** Br. Obstet. Gynaecol 104:1024-1092.

109- De-Bruijn H.W., Ten-Hoor K.A., Krans M., and Vander-Zee A.C. 1997 **Risinf Serum Values of β - Subunit Human Chorionic Gonadotropin (hCG)in Patients with Progressive vulvar Carcinomas** Br.J.cancer 75:1217-1218.

110- Syrigos K.N., Fyssas I.,Konstandoulakeis M.M. Harvington K.J.,Popadapouls S. et al. 2001 **Beta Human Chorionic Gonadotropin Concentration in Serum of Patients with Pancreatic Adenocarcinoma**.Gut 42:88-91.

111- Grow ford R.A., Iles R.K. Carter P.G., Caldwell C.J., Shepherd J.H. ,and Chard T. 1998 **The Prognostic Significance of Beta Human Chorionic Gonadotropin and Its Metabolites in Women with Cervical Carcinoma**. J. clin pathal 51:685-688.

112-Schulter E.M. Mulder C., Van-Kamp G.J., and Keneman S.P., 1997 **The Beta–Core Fragment Chorionic Gonadotropin :Biochemical background and Clinical Application** . Anticancer Res., 17:1255-1272.

113- Schwarz R.U., Petzoldt B., Waldschmidt. et.al., 1997 UGP **A Tumor Marker of Gynecologic and Breast Malignancies Specificity and Sensitivity in Pretherapeutic Patients and the Influence of Hormonal Substitutions on the Expression of UGP** .Anti Cancer Res 17:3041-3045.

114- Acevedo H.F., Krichevsky A., Campbell -Acevedo E.A., Galyon J.C. ,Buffo M.J., and Hartsock R.J. 1992 **Flow Cytometry Methods for the Analysis of Membranes Associated Human Chorionic Gonadotropin , Its subunits, and Fragments on Human cancer cells**, Cancer 69:1818-1828.

115- Acevodo H.F. ,Tong J.Y. and Hartsock R.J. 1995 **Human Chorionic Gonadotropin-beta Subunit Gene Expression in Cultured Human Fetal and Cancer Cells of Different Types and Origins.** cancer 76:1467-1475.

116- Sztumowicz M.SlodKowsta J. Zych J., Rudzinski P., Sakowicz A., Rowinskas 1999 **Frequency and Clinical Significance of Beta Subunit Human Chronic Gonadotropin Expression in Non-small lung Cancer Patients** tumor Biol 20:99-104.

117-Doi F. , Chi D.J., Charuwork B.B., Conrad A.J. Russel J. Morton D.L. 1996 **Detection of ß- Human Chorionicgonadotropin mRNA as a Marker for Coetaneous Malignant Melanoma**. Imt. J. cancer 65:454-459.

118- Lazar V., Diez S.G., Laurent A., Giovanrandi I., Radvanyi F., Chopin D., Bidaart J.M. Bellet D. and Vidaud M. 1995 **Expression of Human Chorionic Gonadotropin ß Subunit Genes in Superficial and Invasive Bladder Carcinoma**. cancer res. 55:3735-3738.

119- Regelson W. 1995 **Have We Found the (Definitive Cancer Biomarker)? The Diagnostic and Therapeutic Implication of Human Chorionic Gonadotropin Beta Expression as a Key to Malignancy.** Cancer 76:1299-1301.

120- Bhalang K., Kafrawy A.H., and Miles D.A. 1999 **Immunohistochemical Study of the Expression of Human Chorionic Gonadotropin Beta in Oral of Sequamous Cell Carcinoma** cancer 85:757-762.

121- Yokotan T. Koizumi T., Tamiguchi R., Nakagawa T., Isobet., et.al. 1997 **Expression of Alpha and Beta Genes of Human Chorionic Gonadotropin in Lung Cancer**. Int.J. cancer 71:539-544.

122- Bieche I,, Lazer V., Nogues C., Poynand I., Giovangrand Y., Bellet D. et.al. 1998 **Prognostic Value of Chorionic Gonadotropin Beta Gene Transcripts in Human Breast Carcinoma Clin.** Cancer Res 4:671-676.

123-Dirhnofer S., Koessler P., Ensinger C., Feichtingerl T., Madersbacher S., and Berger P., 1999 **Production of Trophoblastic Hormones by Transitional Cell Carcinoma of the Bladder Association to Tumor Stage and Grade**. Hum Pathol 29:377-382.

124- Piecioli M., Gamberi B., Pasquinelli G., Poggi S., Ascani S. et.al. 2000. **Beta hCG Aberrant Expression in Primary Mediastinal Large ß-Cell Lymphoma**. Am J. Surg pathol 23:717-721.

125- Acevedo H.F., Hartsockk R.J. 1996 **Metastic Phenotype Correlation with High Expression of Membranes Chorionic Gonadotropin in vivo**. Cancer 78:2388-2399.

126- Gebauer G., Muller-Ruchholtz W. 1997 **Tumor Marker Concentration in Normal and Malignant Tissue of Colorectal Cancer Patients and their Prognostic Relevance**. Anti cancer Res. 17:2731-2734.

127- Walker R.A. 1978 **Significance of ß- subunit hCG Demonstrated in Breast Carcinoma by the Immunoperoxidase Technique** J. clin pathol. 31:245-249.

128- Mohabeer J. Buckly C.H., and fox H. 1983 **An Immunohistochemical Study of the Incidence and Significance of Human Chorionic Gonadotrophin Synthesis by Epithelial Ovarian Neoplasms.** Gynecol oncol. 16:78-84.

129- Oyasu R. Nan L., SmithD.P., and Kawanata H. 1994 **Human Chorionic Gonadotropin β-Subunit Synthesis by Undifferentiation Urothelial carcinoma with syncytiophoblastic differentiation.** Arch. Pathol. Lab. Med 118:715-717.

130- Campo E., Palacin A., Benasco C. Quesada E., and Cardesa A. 1987 **Human Chorionic Gonadotrophin in Colorectal Carcinoma**. Cancer 59:1611-1617.

131- Yakeishi Y., Mori M., and Enjoji M. 1990 **Distribution of β-human Chorionic Gonadotropin –Positive Cells, in Non Cancerous Gastric Mucosa and in Malignant Gastric Tumors** cancer 66:695-701.

132- Collins R.J. and wong L.C. 1989 **Adenocarcinoma of the Uterine Cervix with βhCG Production: A case report and review of the literature.** Gynecol. Oncol 33:99-107

133- Morinaga S., Yamaguchi M., Watanabe I., Kasai M., Ojima M., and Sasano N. 1983 **An immunocytochemical Study of Hepatablastoma Producing Human Chorionic Gonadoropin.**

134- Buckly C.H. and Fox H. 1979 **An Immunohistochemical Study of the Significance of hCG Secretion by Large Bowel Adenocarinoma** .J.clin pathol 32:368-372.

135- Iles R.K. and Chard T. 1989 **Immunochemical Analysis of the Human Chorionic Gondotropin Like Material Secreted by Normal and Neoplastic Urothlial Cells.** J. mol Endocrinol 2:107-112.

136- Yoshimoto Y., Wolfsen A.R., and Odell W.D. 1979 **Human Chorionic Gonadotropin like Material :presence in normal human tissue** Am.J.Obstet .Gynecol 134:729-733.

137- Braunstein G.D., Kamdar V.,and Rosor J., Swomina than N., and Wade M.E. 1979 **Widespread Distribution of a Chorionic Gonadotropin – like Substance in Normal Human Tissue.** J. clin Endocrial Metab 49:917-925.

138- Gillott D.J., Iles R.K, and chard T 1996 **The Effects of Beta Human Chorionic Gonadotrophin on the Invitro Growth of Bladder Cancer Cell lines** Br. J. cancer 73:323-326.

139- Muckherjee K., and Das S.A. 1984 **Placental Glycoprotein , Human Chorionic Gonadotropin as a Growth Stimulant of Murine Tumor Cells.** IRCS med Sci :12 1101-1102.

140- Melmed S. . and Braunstien G.D. 1983 **Human Chorionic Gonadotropin Stimulated Proliferation of Nb2 rat Lymphoma cell** J. clin. Endocrinol. Metab. 1068-1070.

141-Zygmunt M. ,Hahn D., Munstedt K., Bischof P. Lana U. 2000 **Invasion of Cytotrophoblastic JEG.3 Cells is stimulated by hCG in Vitro.** Placenta 19:587-593.

142-Acevedo H.F. Raikow R.B., Powell J.E., and Stevens V. 1987 **Effects of Immunization Against Human Choriogondotropin on the Growth of Transplanted Lewis Lung Carcinoma and Spontaneous Mammary Adenocarcinoma in Mice**: Cancer Detect Prev (Suppl 1): 477-486.

143- Triozzi P.L. , Gochnour D., Martin E.W., and Aldrich W. et. al. 1994 **Clinical and Immunological Effects of Synthetic Beta Human Chorionics Vaccine**. Int J. Oncol 5:1447-1453.

144- Syner L., Woo D., Triozzi P.L. ,and Stevens V., **Synthetic Hormone /Growth Factor Subunit Vaccine with Application to Anti-fertility and Cancer** . In:Powell M.F., and Newman M.J., editors Vaccine Design :the Subunit Approch. New York: plenum Publishing Corp 1995, P907-930.

145- Dufau M.L., Pock R., Neubarer A., Catt K.J. 1976 **Vitro Bioassay of LH in Human Serum: Assay** .J Clin Endocrinol Metab. 42:958-969.

146- Van Damme M.P., Robertson D.M., and Dicz Falusy E. 1974 **An improved in Vitro Bioassay Methods for Measuring Luteinzing Hormone (LH) Activity Using Mouse Leydig Cell Proportions Action**. Endocrinol 77:655-671.

147- Jia X.C., Olkawa M., Bo M., Tanaka T., et.al. 1991 **Expression of Human Luteinizing Hormone (LH) Receptor Interaction with LH and Chorionic Gonadotropin from Human but not Equine, rate and Ovine Species Mol.** Endocrinol 5:759-768.

148- Vaitukaitis J.L.,Braunstien G.D., and Ross G.T. (1972) **Radioimmunoassay Which Specifically Measures Human chorionic Gonadotropin in the presence of Human Luteinizing Hormone** Am J. Obstet Gynecol 113:751-758.

149- Segaloff D.L. ,Sprengel R., Nikolics K., and Accoli M. **Structure of the Lutropin Choriogondotropin receptor**. In Clark J.H(e.) Recent Progress in Hormone Research Vol. 46, A academic Press, INC. San Diego, 1990 , P261-303.

150- Ji T.H., Grossmann M., and Ji J.G. 1998 **G Protein -Coupled Receptors 1.Diversity of Receptor Ligand Interaction**. J. Biol. Chem, 273:17299-17302.

151- Herrlick A., Kuhn B., Grosse R.et.al. 1996 **Involvement of Gs and Gi Proteins in Dual Coupling of the LH Hormone Receptor to Adenyl Cyclase and Phospholipase** C.J. Biol .chem 271:16764-16772.

152- Gudermann T., Birnhaumer M., and Birnbaumer L. 1992 **Evidence for Dual Coupling of the Murine Luteinizing Hormone Receptor to Adenyl Cyclase and Phosphinositide Break Down and Ca^{+2} Mobilization** J. Biol Chem 267:4479-4488.

153- Ekstrom R.C., and Hunzicker D.M. 1989 **Homologous Desensition of Ovarian LH/hCG Receptor Responsive Adenyl Cyclase is Dependent Upon GTP**. Endocrinology 124:956-963.

154- Segaloff D.L., and Ascoli M. 1993 **The Lutropin / Choriogonadotropin Receptor 4 Years Later** Endocr Rev. 14:324-347.

155- Dias , J.A. 1992 **Recent Progress in Structure Function and Molecular Analysis of the Pituitaryl Placental Glycoprotein Hormone Receptors** .Biochem Biophys Acta. 1135:278-294.

156- Bruch R.C., Thotakura N.R., and Bahl O.P. 1986 **The Rat Ovarian Lutropin Receptor: Purification, Hormone Binding Properties, and Subunit Composition**. J. Biol. Chem. 261:9450-9460.

157- Dattatreyamurty B., Rathnam P., and Saxena B.B., 1983 **Isolation of the Luteinzing Hormone -Chorionic Gonadotropin Receptor in High Yield from Bovine Corpora Lutea Molecular Assembly and Oligomeric Nature**. J., Biol Chem. 258:3140-3158.

158- Pandian M.R., and BaHl O.P. 1977 **Labeling of Bovine Corpus Luteal Membranes Human Chorionic Gonadotropin or Luteinzing Hormone (hCG/LH) Receptor and its Purification and Properties** Arch. Bioch. Bioph 182:420-436.

159- Koo Y.B., Ji I., Slaughter R.G., and Ji T.H., 1991 **Structure of the LH Receptor Gene and Multiple Exone of the Coding Sequence** Endocrin 128:2297-2310.

160- Loosfelt H. Misrahi M., Atger M. et.al. 1989 **Cloning and Sequencing of Porcine LH-hCG receptor CDNA: variants lacking transmembrance domine**. Science 245:525-528.

161- Thomas D.M., and Segaloff D.L. 1994 **Hormone Binding Properties and Glycoslation Pattern of a Recombinnant form of the Extracellular Domain of the LH/CG-R Expressed in Mammalian Cells** .Endocrin 135:1902-1912.

162- Hong S.,Phang T., Ji I., and Ji T.H. 1998 **The Amino Terminal Regions of the Lutaining Hormonal Choriogonadotrophin Receptor Contacts Both Subunits of Human Choriogonadotropin I-Mutational Analysis** J. Biol .chem 273:13835-13840.

163- Kanada M., Jablonka S.A.,Sato A. et.al 1999 **Genetic Fusion of an Alpha -Subunit Gene to the Follicle Stimulating Hormone and Chorionic Gonadotropin Beta Subunit Genes :Production of a bifunctional Protein** .Mol Endocrinol 13:1873-1881.

164- Bhowmick N., Huang J., Puett D., Isaacs N. W., and Laphthorn A.J., 1996 **Determination of Residues Important in Hormone Binding to the Extracellular Domain of the Luteinizing Hormone /Chorionic Gonadotropin Receptor by site- Directed Mutagenesis and Modeling**. Mol Endocrine .10:1147-1159.

165- Nagayama Y., Wadsworth H.L. Russo D., Seto P., and Rapoprt B., 1991 **Thyrotropin Luteinizing Hormone/ Chorionic Gonadotropin Receptor**

Extracellular Domain Chimera as Probes for Thyrotrophic receptor Function. Proc Natl Aced Sci USA 88:902-905.

166- Roche P.C. Ryan R.J. and McCormick D.J. 1992 **Identification of Hormone Binding Regions of the Luteinizing Hormone Human Chorionic Gonadotropin Receptor Using Synthetic Peptides.** Endocrinol 131:268-274.

167- Davis D.P., Rozell T.G., Liu X., Segaloff D.L.1997 **The Six N-Linked Carbohydrates of the lutropin/ Choriogonadotropin Receptor are not Absolutely Required for Correct Folding, Cell Surface Expression, Hormone Binding or Signal Transduction.** Mol. Endocriol 11:550-562.

168- Braun T., Schofield P-R., and Sprengel R. 1991 **Amino-Terminal Leucine -Rich Repeats in Gonadotropin Receptors Determine Hormone Selectivity** EMBO J. 10:1885-1890.

169- Kobe B., and Deisenhofer J. 1994 **The Lucien Rich Repeat :A Versatile Binding Motif.** Trends Biochem Sci. 19:415-421.

170- Kobe B., and Deiesenhofer J 1995 **A Structural Basis of the Interaction Between Lucien -Rich Repeats and Protein Ligands.** Nature 374:183-186.

171- Ji T.H., Murdoch W.J. and Ji I 1995 **Activation of Membranes Receptors** Endocrine 3:187-194.

172- Moyle W.R., Campbell R.K., Raos N.V. et.al. 1995 **Model of Human chorionic Gonadotropin and Lutropin Receptor Interaction that Explains Signal Transduction of the Glycoprotein Hormones** J. Biol. Chem .270:20020-20031.

173- Phang T., Kunda G., Hong S., Ji I., and J. T., 1998 **The Amino Terminal Region of the Luteinizing Hormonal Choriogondotropin Receptor Contacts Both Subunits of Human Choriogonadotropin II Photo affinity Labeling** J., Biol Chem 273:13841-13847.

174- Mcfarland K.C., Sprengel R., Phillips H.S., et.al. 1989 **Lutropin - Choriogonadotropin Receptor: An Unusual Member of the G Protein-Coupled Receptor Family.** Science 245:494-499.

175- Jiang X., Dreano M., Buckler D.R.,et.al 1995 **Structural Predictions for the Ligand -Binding Region of Glycoprotein Hormone Receptors and the Nature of Hormone Receptor Interactions.** Structure 3:1341-1353.

176- Hong S., Ji I., Ji T. 1999 . **The β-Subunit of Human Choriogonadotropin Interacts with the Exodomine of the Luteinizing Hormone /Choriogondotropin Receptor and Changes Its Interaction with the α -Subunit.** Mol Endocrinol 13:1285-1294.

177- Ji I., Pan Y., Lee Y., Phang T., and Ji T.H 1995 **Receptor Binding Dependent Structural Changes in Human Choriogonadotropin :photochemical inter subunit cross linking** .Endocrine 3:907-911.

178- Reshef E., Lei Z.M., Rao C., Pridham D.D. et.al. 1990 **The Presence Gonadotropin Receptors in nonpregnant Human Uterus, Human Placenta, Fetal Membranes, and Decidua J.** clin Endocrinol &Metab 70:421-430.

179- Lei Z., Toth P., Rao C., Pridham D.1993 Noval **Coexpression of Human Chorionic Gonadotropin (hCG/Human Luteinizing Hormone Receptors and their Ligand hCG in Human Fallopian Tubes.** J. Clin Endocrinol & Metab 77:863-872.

180-Rao C. Li X. ,Toth , Lei Z. M., and Cook V.D. 1993 **Noval Expression of Functional Hormone Chorionic Gonadotropin /Luteinizing Humane Receptors Gene in Human Umbilical Cords** . J Clin Endocrinol & Metab 77:1706-1714.

181- Rao C. 1996 **The Beginning of a New Area in Reproductive Biology and Medicine :Expression of Low levels of Functional Luteinizing Hormonal Human chorionic Gonadotropin Receptors in Nongonadal Tissue.** J Phsiol Pharmacol 47:41-53

182- Lei Z., Rao C., Kornyei J.L. Licht P., Hiatt E.S. 1993 **Novel Expression of Human Chorionic Gonadotropin /Luteinizing Hormone Receptor Gene in Brain** Endocirnol 132:2262-2270.

183- Meduri G., Charnaux N., Loosfell H., Jolivet A et.l. 1997 **Luteinzing Hormone /Human chorionic Gonadotropin Receptor in Breast Cancer.** Cancer Rech. 57:857-864.

184- Lin J. Lei Z. Lojuns S., Rao C.et al 1994 **Luteinizing Hormone/Human Chorionic Gonadotropin Receptor Gene in Human Endometrial Carcinomas** J.Clin Endocrionol & Metab 79:1483-1491.

185- Huang Z.H., Lei Z., and Rao C. 1995 **Immortalized and Erior Pituitary & T3 Gonadotropes Contain Functional Luteinizing Hormone/Humane Chorionic Gonadotropin Receptors** . Mol Cell Endocrinol 114:217-222.

186- Pabon J.E., Bird J.S., Li X., Huang Z.H. et.al. 1996 **Human Skin Contains Luteinizing Hormone /Chorionic Gonadotropin Receptors** J. Clin Endocrinol & Metab .81:2738-2741.

187- Lei Z.M. ,Reshef E., and Rao C. 1992 **The Expression of Human Chorionic Gonadotrpin Luteinizing Hormone Receptors in Human Endometrial and Myometrial Blood Vessels**. J. Clin Endocrnol & Metab 75:651-659.

188- Kornyel J., Leiz., and Rao C., 1993 **Human Myometrial Smooth Muscle Cells and Human Chorionic Gonadotropin**. Biol Reprod. 49:1149-1157.

189- Ziecik A.J..Stanchev P.D., Tilton J.E., 1986 **Evidence for the presence of Luteinizing Hormonal/ Human Chorionic Gonadotropin Binding Sites in the Porcine Uterus**. Endocrinol .119:1159-1163.

190- Bonnamy P.O. Benhaim A., and Leymaric P. 1989 **Human chorionic Gonadotropin Affects Tissue Levels of Progesterone and Cyclic Adenosine 3,5 Monophosphate in the Metestrus Rat Uterus in Vitro** . Biol Reprod 40:511-516.

191- Menon K. , and Jaffe R.B. 1973 **Chorionic Gonadotropin Sensitive Adenylate Cyclase in Human Placenta**. J Clin Endocrinol & Metab. 36:1140-9.

192- Demeros L.M. Gabbe S.G., Villee C.A., and Greep Ro. 1973 **Human Chorionic Gonadotropin Mediated Glycogenolysis in Human Placental** Villi .Biophys Acta 313:202-210.

193- Wolf A., Henrich I., Benz R., and Lauritzen C. 1985 **Influence of Human Chorionic Gonadotropin and Prostaglandins on the steroid Metabolism of the perfused placenta** Contr Gynecol Obstet 13:162-164.

194- Varangot J. Cedard L., and Yannotti S., 1965 **Perfusion of Human Placenta in Vitro Study of the Biosynthesis of Estrogens.** Am J Obst Gynecol 92:534-547.

195- Rosenberg S. M., and Bhanager A.S. 1984 **Sex Steriod and Human Chorionic Gonadotropin Modulation of in Vitro Prolactin Production by Human Term Decidua**. Am J. Obstet Gynecol 148:461-466.

196- Yuen B.H. Moon Y., Shin D. 1986 **Inhibition of Human Chorionic Gonadotropin Production by Prolactin From Term Human Trophoblast** Am. J. Obstet Gynecol 154:336-340.

197- Lojun S., Bao S., Lei Z.M. , and Rao C. 1997 **Presence of Functional Luteinizing Hormone / Chorionic Gonadotropin (hCG) Receptors in Human Breast Cell Lines:Implications Supporting the Premise that** hCG Protects Women Against Breast Cancer. Biol Reprod 57:1202-1210.

198-Russo J. and Russo I H. 1995 **Hormonally Induced Differentiation :A Novel Approach to Breast Cancer Prevention** J. Cell Biochem 22 (suppl 1.):58-64.

199-Alvarado M.V., Russoo J. ,Alvarado N.E., and Russo I., 1994 **Human Chorionic Gonadotropon inhibits proliferation and Induces Expression of Inhibin in Human breast Epithelial cells in Vitro** .In Vitro Cell &Dev Biol 30A:4-8.

200-lowry O.H.,Resebrough N.J.,Farr A.L. and Randall R.J. 1951 **Protein Measurement with the Folin Reagent** .J. biol. Chem. 193:265-275.

201- Strickland S., and Richards W.G. 1992 **Invasion of the Trophoblast Cells**.Cell 71:355-357.

202- Goustin A.C, Bestsholtz, C., Pfeifer- Ohlsson S., Persson H., Rydnert J. Bywater M et al. 1985 **Coexpression of the sis and myc Proto-oncogene in Developing human Placenta Suggests Autocrine Control of Trophoblast Growth** .Cell 41:301-312.

203- Chassin D. ,.Benifa J.L., Delattre C., fernandez H., Ginist D. , Janneau J., et al. 1994 **Identification of Genes Over Expressed in Tumors Through Preferential Expression Screening in Trophoblast**. Cancer Res. 54:5217-5223.

204- Bennett W. A., Lagoo Deenadayalan S., Whitworth N.S., stopple J. A., Barber W.H. et. Al. 2000 **First -Trimester Human Chorionic Villi Express Both Immuno Regulatory and Inflammatory Cytokines :a role for interleukin-10 in regulating the cytokine network of pregnanancy.** Am. J. Reprod -Immuno 41:70-8.

205-Bonnamy P.J., Benhaim A., Leymarie P. 1990 **Estrous Cycle – Related Change of High Affinity Luteinizing Hormone/ Human Chorionic Gonadotropin Binding Sites in the Rat Uterus.** Endocrinol 126:1264-1269.

206-Bennett J.P,, and Yamamura H.I **Neurotransmitter Hormone, or Drug Receptor Binding Methods** .In Yamamura H.I., Enna S.J., Kuhar M.J., (eds) Neurotransmitter Receptor Binding (2ed). Raven Press New York 1985 P61-89..

207-Shao K., Balasubramania S.V., Pope C.M., and Bahl O.P., 1998 **Effect of Individual N- Glycosyl chains in the ß-Subunit on the conformation of Human Choriogonadotropin** Mol cell Endocrinol.146:39-48.

208-Bellisario R., and Bahl O.P. 1975 **Human chorionic Gonadotropin V. Tissue Specificity of Binding and Partial Characterization of Soluble Human Chorionic Gonadotropin –Receptor Complexes** J. Biol .chem. 250:3837-3844.

209-Rao C.V., **Receptors for Gonadotropins in Human Ovaries** In:Muldoon T.G., Mahesh V.B., Peez Ballester B., (eds) Recent Advances in Fertility Research, Part A. New York:Liss; 1982,P123-135.

210-Marsh J.M. 1976 **The Role of Cyclic AMP in Gonadal Steroidogensis**. Biol Reprod .14:30-53.

211-Huhtaniemi L.T., and Catt K.J. 1981 **Differential Binding Affinities of Rat Testis Luteini Hormone (LH) Receptors for Human Chorionic Gonadotropin Human LH, and Ovine LH.** Endocrinol. 108:1931-1938.

212-Wittliff J.L., **Hormone and Growth Factor Receptor** In: Donegan W.L. and Spratte J.S. (ed) Cancer of the Breast, 4ed Philadelphia:w.B. Saunders Co. 1995 pp 346-369.

213-Janson P.O. 1975 **Effects of the Luteinizing Hormone on Blood in the Follicular Rabbit Ovary as Measured by Radioactive Microsphers**. Acta Endocrinol 79:122-133.

214- Willtbank M.c., Gallagher K.P., Dysko R.C., Keyes P.L., 1089 **Regulation of Blood Flow to the Rabbit Corpus Luteum: Effects of Estradiol and Human chorionic Gonadotropin** Endocrinol. 124:605-611.

215-Korenman S.G., Krall J.F., 1977 **The Role of Cyclic AMP in the Regulation of Smooth Muscle Cell Contraction in the Uterus** Biol Reprod. 16:1-17.

216-Joshi S.G., 1983. **Progestin Regulated Proteins of the Human endometrium**. Sem Reprod Endocrinol 1:21-36.

217-Jacobs S., and Cuatrecasas P. **Problems in Studying Hormone Receptor Binding** .In Jacob J (ed.) Advances in Pharmacology and Therapeutics Vol.1 Pergamon , New York 1979 PP.215-222.

218-Jacobs S.Chang K.J., and Cuatercases P.1975 **Estimation of Hormone Receptor Affinity by Competitive Displacement of Labeled ligand :Effect of Concentration of Receptor and of Labeled ligand** Biochem . Biophys Res. Commun .66:687-692.

219-Dufau M.L., Ryan D.W., Baukal A. J., and Catt K.J. 1975 **Gonadotropin Receptors: Solubilization and Purification by Affinity Chromatography**. J. Biol chem. 250:4822-4824.

220-Keutmann H.T., 1992 **Receptor. Binding Regions in Human Glycoprotein Hormones** Mol. Cell Endocrinol 86:1-6.

221- Ruddon R.W., Byran A.H., Hanson C.A., Perini F., et. al. 1981 **Characterization of the Intracellular and Secreted Forms of the Glycoprotein Hormone Chorionic Gonadotropin Produced by Human Malignant Cells**. J. Biol chem. 256:5189-5196.

222-Keutmann H.J., M cllory P.J. Bergert E.R., Ryan R.J., 1983 **Chemically Deglycosylated Human Chorionic Gonadotropin Subunits: characterization and biological properties** .Biochemistry 22:3067-3072.

223-Kalyan N.K. and Bahl O.P 1983 **Role of Carbohydrate in Human Chorionic Gonadotropin :Effect of Deglycosylation on the Subunit Interaction and on its in Vitro and in Vivo Biological properties** J. Biol Chem 258:67-74.

224-Ascoli M. Puett D. 1978 **Gonadotropin Binding and Stimulation of Steroidogenesis in Leyding Tumors Cells** Proc Natl Acad Sci USA 75:99-102.

225-Dufau M.L., Charreau E.H. and Catt K.J. 1974 **Characteristics of a Soluble Gonadotropin Receptor From the Rat Testis** J., Biol. Chem 248:6973-76.

226-Haour F., Saxena B.B. 1974 **Characterization and Solubilization Gonadotropin Receptor of Bovine Corpus Luteum** J. Biol chem. 248: 2195-2199.

227-Vutlai Luu Thi M.T., Misrahi M., Houllier A., Jolivet A, Milgrom E.1992 **Variant Form of the Pig Lutropin/ Choriogonadoropin Receptor**. Biochemistry 31:8377-8383.

228-Pandian M.R., Bahl O.P.,and Segal S.J. 1975 **Labeling of LH/CG Receptor in Rat Ovaries** Biochem Biophys. Res. Commun 64:1199-1205.

229-Sexena B.B. **In Methods in Receptor Research** (Blecher M.,ed) Part I, Marcel Dekker New York 1976, P 251-292.

230-LKB Application Note 306.1977 **SDS and Conventional Polyacrymide GEL Electrophoresis with LKB Muitiphor.**

231- Segrest J.P. and Jackson R.C. **In Method In Enzymology** (V.Ginsburg, ed.) Vol XXVIII, Academic press N. Y., 1972, P481.

232- Dubois M., Gilles K.A., Hamilton J.K., Rebers P.A, and Smith F. 1956 **Colorimetric method for determination of sugars and related substance**. Anal. Chem. 28:350-356.

233- Garfin D.E. In Method in Enzymology (Dentschr M. P., ed) Vol 182, Academoc Press Inc., 1990, P459.

234- Igarashi S., Minegishi T., Nakamura K., Nakamura M., et.al. 1994 **Functional Expression of Recombinant Human Luteinizing Hormone Human Choriogonadotropin Receptor,** Biochem Biohys Res. Commun. 201:248-256.

235- Mc farland K.C. Sprengel R., Phillips H.S., Kohler M. et.al. 1989 **Lutropin –Chorio Gonadoropin Receptor: An Unusual Member of the G-Protein Coupled Receptor Family**. Science 245:494-499.

236- Rosemblit N., Ascoli M, Segaloff D.L. 1988 **Characterization of a Antiserum to the Rat Luteinizing Hormone/Chorionic Gonadotropin Receptor**. Endocrinology 123: 2284-2290.

237- Loosfelt H., Misrahi;M. Atger M., Salesse R., et al. 1989 **Cloning and Sequencing of Porcine LH/CG Receptor CDNA: Variants Lacking Transmembrance Domain** .Science 245:525-528.

238- Minegishi T., Nakamura K., Takakura Y., Miyamato K., Hasegawa Y., Igarashi M. 1990 **Cloning and Sequencing of Human LH/CG Receptor CDNA**. Biochem Biophys Res Commun. 172:1049-1054.

239- Rodrignez M.C., Segaloff D.L. 1990 **The Orientation of the Lutropin/Choriogonadotropin Receptor as Revealet by Site-Specific Antibodies** Endocrinology 127:674-681.

240- Hipkin R.W, Sanchez. Yague J., Ascoli M. 1992 **Identification and Characterization of a Luteinizing Hormone Chorionic Gonadotropin (LH/CG)Receptor Precursor in a Human Kidney Cell Line Stably Transfected with the Rat Luteal LH/CG Receptor Complementary DNA** Mol Endocrinol 6:2210-2218.

241- Ascoli M., Segaloff D.L. 1989 **On the Structure of the Luteinizing Hormonal/ Chorionic Gonadotropin Receptor**. Endocr Rav. 10:27 – 44.

242- Pataja –Repo U.E., Merz W.E. Rajaniemi H.J. 1991 **Significance of the Glycan Moiety of the Rat Ovarian Luteinzing Hormone/Chorionic Gonadotropin and Human CG for Receptor- Receptor – Hormone Interaction**. Endocrinology 128:1209-1217.

243- Ji I., Slaughter R.G., Ji T.H. 1990 **N-Linked Oligosaccharides are not Required for Hormone Binding of the Lutropin Receptor in a Leyding Tumor cell Line and Rat Granulosa Cell**. Endocrinology 127:494-406.

244- Zhang R., Tsai Morris C.H., Kitamura M., Buczko E., Dufau M.L. 1991 **Changes in Binding Activity of Lutenizing Hormone Receptors by Site Direct Mutagenesis of Potential Glycosylation Sites.** Biochem Biophys Res Commun 181:804-808.

245- Liu X., Davis D., Segaloff D.L. 1993 **Disruption of Potential Glycosylation Sites for N-Linked Glycosylation Does not Impair Hormone Binding to the Lutropin /Choriogonadotropin (LH/CG) Receptor if Asn 173 is left intact**. J Biol chem. 268:1513-1516.

246- Freifrlder D(ed). **Physical Biochemistry, Application to Biochemistry and Molecular Biology** 2th(ed.) San Fransico, W.H. Freeman and Company, 1982.

247- Silvestien R.M., Basster G.C., Morril T.C. eds. **Spectrophotometric Identification of Organic Compounds** New York. Joun Wiley & Sons 1981.

248-Ascoli M.1982 **Internalization and Degradation of Receptor-Bound Human Choriogonadotropin in Leyding Tumor Cells Fate of the Hormone Subunits** J.Biol. Chem 257:13306 -13311.

249-Tsavaris P.Vonorta K. ,Tsoutsos H.,Kozatsani –Halividi D. et al 1993 **Carcinoembryonic Antigen (CEA), α -Feto-Protein, CA 19-9 and CA-125 in Advanced Colorectal Cancer (ACC)**. In J Biol Markers. 8:88-93.

250-Chevinsky A.H. 1991 **CEA in Tumor of Other Than Colorectal Origin** .Semin Surg Oncol .7:162-166.

251-DiSaia P. ,Haverback B.J., Dyce B.J. Marrow C.P 1975 **Carcinoembryonic Antigen in Patients with Gynecologic Malignancies.** Am J Obstet Gynecol .121:159-163.

252-Barrelet V., Mack J.P. 1975 **Variations of the Carcinoembryonic Antigen Level in the Plasma of Patients with Gynecologic Cancers During Therapy** . Am. J. Obstet Gynecol 121:164-168.

253-Schwartz P.E., Chambers S.K., Chambers J.T., et.al 1987. **Circulating Tumor Markers in the Monitoring of Gynecologic Malignancies**. Cancer 60:353-361.

254-Tuxen M.K., Soletormos G., Domber-nowsky G.1995 **Tumor Marker in the Management of Patients with Ovarian Cancer**. Cancer Treat Rev 21:215-245.

255-Stall K.E., Martin E.W. 1981 **Plasma Carcinoembryonic Antigen Levels in Ovarian Cancer Patients :A Chart Review and Survey of Published Data**. J Reprod Med. 26:75-82.

256-Cohen C., Shulman G., Budgeon L.R. 1982 **Endocervical and Endometrial Adenocarcinma :A Immunoperoxidase and Histochemical Study**. Am. J. Surg. Pathol .6:151-156.

257-Van Nagell J. R., Donaldson E.S., Gay E.C., et.al 1979 **Carcinoembryonic Antigen in Carcinoma of the Uterine Cervix. Tissue Localization and correlation with plasma Antigen Concentration**. Cancer 44:944-984.

258-Bychkov V., Rothman M., Bardawill W.A 1983 **Immunocytochemical Localization of Carcinoembryonic Antigen(CEA), Alpha –Fetoprotein (AlP), and Human Chorinic Gonadotropin (hCG) in Cervical Neoplasia** Am. J. Clin .Pathol. 79:414-420.

259-Berbec H., Paszkawska A., Siwek B., Gradziel K., Cybulski M. 1999 **Total Serum Sialic Acid Concentration as a Supporting Marker of Malignancy in Ovarian Neoplasia** Eur.J. Gynaec. Oncol 6:389-392.

260-Nathanson L., Fishman W.H 1971 **New Obersation on the Regan Isoenzyme of Alkaline Phosphatase in Cancer Patients** Cancer 27:1388-1397.

261-Kellen J.A., Bush R.S., Malkin A., 1976 **Placenta –Like Alkaline Phosphates in Gynecological Cancer** .Cancer Res.36:269-271.

262-Nollwen E.J., Pollet D.E., Schelstraete J.B., et al. 1985 **Human Placental Alkalinee Phosphatase in Benign and Malignant Ovarian Neoplasia** .**Cancer** Res.45:892-902.

263-Shetty P.A., Damle S.R. and Shahane A.I 1985 **Clinical Significance of heat labile regan isoenzyme variant in Hodgkin's disease**. Cancer 55:605-607.

264-Milne D.B., **Trace Elements in Tietz Text Book of Clinical Chemistry** 3rd ed. W.B. Sannders Company P.1030 -1031, 1999.

265-WHO **Trace Element in Human Nutrition and Health** 1996.

266-Malk K.L., Bhardway S.D., and Seigh P.P 1989 **Diagnostic and Prognostic Value to Serum Zinc, Copper in Different Type of Malignancies** .Excerpta Medica.

267- **Bates M. Bronchial Carcinoma an Integrated Approach for Diagnosis and Management Springer-Verlag Berlin Heidlberg**, New Youk P129,1984.

268- Henderson J.Shuskik C., Kremer R. and et al 1989 **Circulating Levels of Parathyroid Hormone –Like Peptide in Patients with Malignancy and Hypercalcemia** .Clin Oncol Suppl.8

269- Rieke J.W.Donaldson S.S.,and Horning S.J 1989 **Hypercalcemia and Vitamin D Metabolism in Hodgkin's Disease Cancer** 63:1700-1707.

270- Waxman J.1990 **Hypercalcaemia –New Mechanism for Old Observation** Br.J. Cancer 61:647-648.

271- Bondy P.K., and Gitby E.D. 1982 **Endocrine Function in Small Cell Undifferentiated Carcinoma of the Lung**. Cancer 50:2147-2153.

272- Kaplan L.A., and Pesce A.H. eds.**Clinical Chemistry -Theory , Analysis and Correlation** 2nd (ed.) Mosby Company ST Louis 1989 P924-930.

273- **Valery's Practical Clinical Biochemistry** Gowenlock A.H., McMurray J.R., and Mclauchlan D.M (eds) 6th(ed.) Heinmann Medical book,London 1988.

274- Katopodis N., Hirashaut Y., Nancy L.G. and Stock C.C 1982 **Lipid Associated Sialic Acid Test for the Detection of Human Cancer**.Cancer Res 42:5270-5275.

275- Saif Allah P.H. **Biochemical Studies on Prolactin and some Tumor Markers in Breast Cancer** Ph. D Thesis .Colleg of Science, Baghdad Univ .2000.

276- Landenson J.H., ,and Bower G.N 1973 **Free Calcium in Serum Clin** .Chem. 19:575-582.

277- Gordan G.S., Fitzpatrick M.E., and Lubich W.P. 1967 .**Identification of Osteolytic Sterols in Human Breast Cancer** .Trans .Ass. Amer. Physocians 80:183-186.

278- Greaves M., Ibbotson K.J., Atkins D. and Martin T.J. 1980 **Prostaglandins as Mediators of Bone Resorption in Renal and Breast Tumors**. Clin Sci 58:201-204.

279- Tashjian A.H., Voeikel E.F., Lazzaro M., Bosma T., and Levine L. 1987 **Tumor Necrosis Factors stimulates Bone Resorption in Mouse Calvaria Prostoglandin –Mediated Mechanism**. Endocrinology 120:270-275.

280- Lorenzo J.A., Quinton J., Sousa S.,and Raisz L.G 1986 Effect of DNA and Prostaglandin Synthesis Inhibitor on the Stimulation of Bone Resorption by **Epidermal Growth Factor in Fetal Rat Long- bone Cultures** J. Clin Invest 77:1897-19001.

281- Sato K.,Fujll Y., Kasond K., and et al., 1989 **Parathyroid Hormone –Related Protein and Interleukin I a Synergism Stimulate Bone Resorptio in Vitro and Increase the Serum Calcium Concentration in Mice in Vivo**. Endocrinol 124:2172-2176.

www.ingramcontent.com/pod-product-compliance
Lightning Source LLC
Chambersburg PA
CBHW060008210526
45170CB00017B/1979